Chair Yoga Mastery

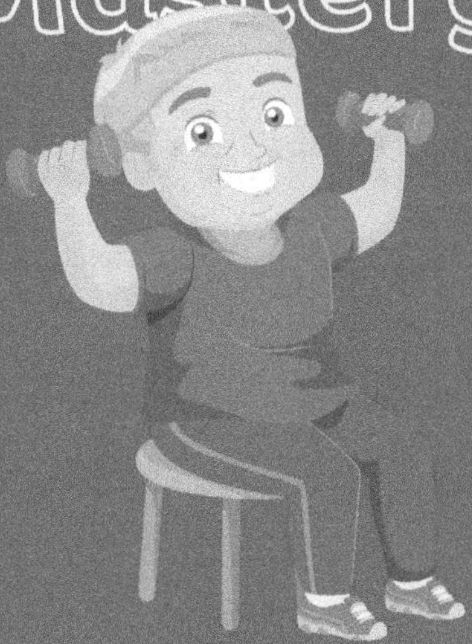

Effortless Senior Wellness in 10 Minutes a Day!

Christopher E. Alber

Chair Yoga Mastery

Effortless Senior Wellness in 10 Minutes a Day!

By

Christopher E. Alber

Table of contents

Introduction

We frequently find ourselves disregarding the demands of our bodies and minds in the midst of life's hustle and bustle. This neglect can have a negative impact on our energy and wellbeing, especially for those of us who have accepted the golden years of 60 and beyond. Fear not, though, for this book has a shortcut to wellbeing that only takes a few minutes of your day to complete. "Chair Yoga Mastery: Effortless Senior Wellness in 10 Minutes a Day" is yours to explore.

Imagine that it is a peaceful morning and that the sun is shining softly through your windows. A feeling of serenity envelopes you as you drink your morning tea. You're about to embark on a self-care adventure that will completely alter how you live out your senior years. Though it can seem like a pipe dream, becoming flexible, active, and balanced is closer than you might imagine.

Allow me to tell you a tale. Meet Sarah, a young and energetic soul who recently turned 65. She saw a decrease in her flexibility and less energy to engage in her favorite pastimes as the years went by. She was a little discouraged and questioned whether she should just accept this as an inevitable byproduct of aging. But later, a chance meeting caused everything to alter.

Sarah met Jane, a bright woman in her 70s, at a local community event one sunny afternoon. Jane's energy and grace enthralled Sarah. Jane revealed the solution: chair yoga. Sarah was intrigued and made the decision to try it. She soon realized that chair yoga was more than just poses; it was a means for her to find the potential of her body.

Sarah discovered that she was gradually rediscovering her flexibility as she immersed herself in her chair yoga practice. Years of stress began to slip away with each stretch, leaving her feeling liberated. Her spirit was energized as well as relaxed by the breathing exercises. Her heart was pounding in the best manner imaginable after the quick but effective cardiovascular exercises, which also increased her level of overall vitality.

Sarah's experience is not unusual. Numerous people like her are enjoying the beauty of chair yoga every day. What's best? It only takes ten minutes. That is far less time than it takes to make your morning coffee or read the news. You are starting a transforming journey—one that honors your body, your spirit, and your progress through the years—by devoting these priceless times to yourself.

We shall examine the science and practice of chair yoga on the pages that follow. Myths will be debunked, postures created specifically for your requirements will be explored, and you'll be led through a thorough practice that addresses flexibility, balance, strength, and relaxation. We'll also share true accounts of people like Sarah, whose lives have been improved by chair yoga.

Are you prepared to start along the road to uncomplicated senior wellness? Allow this book to serve as your inspiration, guidance, and companion. You can start a life-changing adventure by investing just 10 minutes a day in it. It will not only improve your physical health but also give your life a greater feeling of joy and vigor. Let's begin the journey together right now.

Chapter 1

The Power of Chair Yoga

Understanding the Benefits

Imagine this in your mind's eye for a moment: a tranquil park where a calming symphony is created by the distant buzz of life and the soft rustling of leaves. A group of elderly people congregate in the center of the park, their faces beaming with grins and brimming with life. They're here for chair yoga, not a marathon or a strenuous workout.

Meet James, a 68-year-old retired man who once had reservations about yoga. He believed it to be a privilege of the adaptable and the young and a completely unrelated activity to his everyday life. But he learned about chair yoga one day while conversing with a buddy at the neighborhood senior center. James's interest piqued, he made the decision to try it, and that choice resulted in a major change in his life.

James was welcomed by Anna, the welcoming teacher, as he entered his first chair yoga session. She informed the participants that this activity was created to offer joy rather than stress and was adapted to their capacities. James sat down in his chair as the meeting got underway, unsure of what to anticipate. First, he was surprised to learn that chair yoga was more than just doing positions that made him look like a pretzel; it was also about embracing movement, breathing, and awareness in a way that was comfortable for his body.

Imagine now the advantages that James experienced. He saw his muscles becoming more flexible, his joints becoming more fluid, and his posture getting better with each session. His body responded favorably to the mild stretches and motions, which eased the stiffness that had developed over the years. What was even more amazing was the mental adjustment he went through. He experienced a sense of peace that he hadn't experienced in a long time as he coordinated his breathing with his actions.

James's experience is but one of many. There are countless advantages to chair yoga, and they can also change your life. Let's explore these advantages in greater detail to reveal the full power of chair yoga.

The Advantage of Flexibility

Our bodies alter as we progress through life. Movements that formerly appeared effortless may become difficult when joints get stiff and muscles lose their flexibility. Chair yoga offers a mild yet powerful remedy for this. The primary goals of chair yoga are to lengthen and stretch the muscles, improve joint mobility, and broaden the range of motion.

Imagine being able to reach for products on high shelves or tie your shoelaces without thinking twice. Through chair yoga, these seemingly insignificant duties can become sources of empowerment. The poses and stretches, which have been modified for your sitting position, work in unison to relieve stress, increase flexibility, and encourage fluidity in your movements.

Enhancing Your Body and Mind

The advantages of chair yoga don't just apply to the physical body; they also apply to the mind and spirit. Imagine beginning each day with a peaceful heart and a mind that is full of optimism. The focus on mindfulness and breathing exercises in chair yoga might support you in achieving your goals. You are bringing a strong sense of present into your practice as you move through each pose and time your breath.

Let's pause now and consider Mary's path. She had gone through her fair share of ups and downs by the time she was 70. She frequently felt overwhelmed by life's stresses and health issues. But she found refuge in chair yoga. She discovered a haven from the troubles that had formerly filled her mind with each breath in and breathe out. She was able to develop gratitude and present via the practice, which gave her a renewed sense of resilience as she dealt with the difficulties of life.

Enhancing Coordination and Balance

Have you ever been in awe of a dancer's exquisite movements or a gymnast's unwavering balance? Although you may not have aspirations of performing on a stage, balance and coordination are crucial in day-to-day activities. Chair yoga presents positions that concentrate on enhancing balance, stability, and coordination, enabling you to move confidently through your surroundings.

Imagine proceeding without even a trace of doubt onto a moving bus or down a cobblestone walkway. Your proprioception—the awareness of your body's location and movements—is improved by chair yoga. This improved balance can be a game-changer, lowering your danger of falling and enabling you to fully appreciate life's adventures.

Maintaining Heart Health

Your heart merits your care and attention because it has been pounding steadily since the day you were born. Chair yoga is aware of this, and its cardiovascular exercises are made to maintain the health of your heart without undue strain on your body. You boost your cardiovascular system and enhance blood circulation by making slow, regulated motions that slightly increase your heart rate.

Imagine your heart as a steadfast traveler making their way through life. It has a smoother route thanks to chair yoga, keeping it robust and sturdy. By performing these heart-nourishing exercises, you are not only improving your physical health but also the vigor that powers your daily activities.

A Way to Reduce Stress

Stress frequently enters our lives like an unauthorized guest. The stresses of modern life can damage both the body and the psyche, especially when combined with the difficulties that come with getting older. Here's when the relaxation methods from chair yoga can save the day.

Think of a situation where tension doesn't control your emotions or drain your energies. With chair yoga, you have the resources to manage stress in a kind and efficient way. You're releasing any stress that may have built up over time through guided relaxation and deep breathing. In the midst of life's storms, you are giving yourself the gift of inner peace, a haven of tranquility.

Getting Involved in a Helpful Community
Imagine being a part of a group that supports you, acknowledges your accomplishments, and offers a secure environment for development. In addition to nourishing your own personal

journey, chair yoga also connects you to a community of people who have similar interests and aims.

Take Joan, an 80-year-old who was originally hesitant to sign up for a chair yoga class. But as she sat down and joined in the discussions, she found a group of people who welcomed her with open arms. She felt a sense of belonging she hadn't had in a long time thanks to the laughter, camaraderie, and common will to succeed. Joan found a group of friends through chair yoga who not only helped her restore her physical strength but also brightened her spirits.

a holistic strategy towards wellness

It becomes clear that chair yoga is a holistic method of wellbeing as we peel back the layers of its advantages. It involves more than just bending and stretching; it also involves embracing movement, taking care of your mind, developing resilience, and interacting with a caring community. Chair yoga acknowledges that wellness is a journey that develops through everyday practice and a mindful way of living.

Imagine starting your 10-minute chair yoga exercise each morning with a sense of anticipation, knowing that it will open the door to life, happiness, and wellbeing. You will explore chair yoga's postures, techniques, and the experiences of those whose lives have been impacted by its transformational potential as you progress through the following sections.

Chair yoga is an invitation to appreciate your body and the richness of your senior years by strengthening your flexibility, empowering your mind, fostering balance, and nourishing heart health. Are you prepared to start this adventure, dear reader? Together, let's take the first step.

Overcoming common misconceptions

Imagine a small gathering of elders in a peaceful space with delicate lighting for their first chair yoga class. One of them is Sarah, a retired woman who has heard about yoga's advantages but has never given it any thought for herself. She sinks into her chair as her mind is racing with ideas. Yoga isn't for the young and flexible, right? She muses, "Can I really achieve this?

Sarah's inquiries reveal widespread misconceptions about chair yoga, which have prevented many people from benefiting from its transformational impact. We'll explore these myths in this chapter, dispelling them with actual accounts and information that will give you the courage and zeal to embrace chair yoga.

Misconception 1: Yoga Is Only for Flexible and Young People

If you've ever seen photos of yogis twisting themselves into challenging positions, you might have assumed, "Yoga is only for the super flexible and the young." However, especially when it comes to chair yoga, this couldn't be further from the truth.

Let's meet Robert, a 75-year-old retiree who thought that due to his weak flexibility, yoga was out of his league. He chose to go to a chair yoga class after letting his curiosity win. He found that the exercise was appropriate for him as soon as he got into his chair. Regardless of each student's level of flexibility, the instructor led the class through mild stretches and routines.

Robert's experience demonstrates how flexible chair yoga is. It's about nourishing your body's individual needs and abilities, not about striking Instagram-worthy poses. Chair yoga is created to meet you where you are on your path to wellbeing through seated poses and slow, deliberate movements.

Misconception 2: Seniors shouldn't do yoga due to its intensity

The idea that yoga is physically taxing and unsuited for seniors may arise from the sight of yoga practitioners contorted into pretzel-like poses. But chair yoga is a mild but effective approach to experience yoga's health benefits without putting too much stress on your body.

Take Maria, a 70-year-old who was worried about her strength and endurance. She was concerned that she would find traditional yoga to be too demanding. But when she came across chair yoga, she understood that it provided the ideal balance of activity and relaxation. She was able to practice in a way that respected rather than pushed her body's limits because the poses were adjusted to her sitting position.

The focus of chair yoga is on security and comfort. Developing a sense of wellbeing involves pushing oneself just enough to feel uncomfortable. You'll find that chair yoga is a gentle method to improve strength and flexibility while acknowledging your body's capabilities because it focuses on controlled movements and appropriate alignment.

24

Misconception 3: Chair yoga is not a "real" workout, contrary to popular belief.
Chair yoga could appear too soft to be considered a real workout in a society that frequently associates fitness with strenuous activity. The advantages of chair yoga, however, go far beyond the perspiration and rigor of regular exercise.

Meet 80-year-old Emily, who was accustomed to more strenuous kinds of exercise. She anticipated a simple session when she went to a chair yoga class. She found a practice that worked her muscles, helped her posture, and made her feel re-energized. She was unexpectedly challenged by the balancing and core-strengthening exercises, demonstrating that chair yoga might be a legitimate workout.

The goal of chair yoga is to promote overall health. While chair yoga may not cause you to sweat as much as a high-impact workout would, it activates your muscles, improves flexibility, and supports cardiovascular health in a sustainable and gentle manner.

Misconception 4: Chair yoga is monotonous and boring

Chair yoga may conjure up images of boring or tedious sitting in a chair for extended periods of time. But chair yoga is a dynamic form of exercise that provides a range of positions and motions to keep you interested.

Imagine Lucy, a 68-year-old expecting a sedentary experience from her chair yoga session. She was pleasantly surprised by the variety of exercises, which ranged from easy stretches to more intense ones. The instructor kept the class interesting and fun by introducing inventive twists.

A canvas for discovery is provided by chair yoga. It's about appreciating movement's beauty when confined to a chair. You'll discover fresh methods to exercise your body, stimulate your mind, and set off on a path of self-discovery with each session.

Misconception 5: Chair yoga doesn't connect the mind and body.

Yoga is frequently praised for fostering a connection between the mind and body, but you might wonder if this connection can really be fostered while sitting in a chair. In actuality, chair yoga presents an extraordinary opportunity to develop mindfulness and self-awareness.

Consider John, a 72-year-old who enjoyed meditation but was dubious of chair yoga's capacity to promote awareness. He found in his first session that the slow, purposeful motions and coordinated breathing drew him into the present. He discovered that chair yoga improved both his physical health and his relationship with his body and breath.

The precise and focused movements of chair yoga are what give it its mindfulness component. Breathing in time with each action creates a link between your body and mind that can enhance your sensation of the present and promote calm.

Embracing the Truth: The Inclusivity and Power of Chair Yoga

The experiences of Sarah, Robert, Maria, Emily, Lucy, and John dispel prevalent myths that have prevented people from benefiting from the transformative potential of chair yoga. The exercise overcomes monotony, rigidity, age, and adaptability. It provides a holistic strategy that honors the individuality of your body and promotes your wellbeing.

We'll keep dispelling these myths and illuminating the genuine core of chair yoga as we progress through this book. You'll learn about the wide range of advantages that are waiting for you through stories, insights, and helpful advice. It's time to face the reality: chair yoga is a gift that is available to people of all ages and abilities and is joyful as well as profoundly transforming. So let's put these myths to rest and enter a world of wellness that embraces you for who you are.

Chapter 2

Getting Started Safely

Preparing Your Space

Consider a tranquil area of your home that is ornamented with soothing details and drenched in soft light. This is your sacred space, the blank canvas on which your journey through chair yoga will take shape. To completely embrace the practice of chair yoga, it's important to create a welcoming environment, just as an artist prepares their palette before painting a masterpiece.

Meet Laura, a 62-year-old who at first struggled to set up the ideal setting for her chair yoga sessions. She struggled to fully commit to the exercise since she was kept from doing so by noise and clutter from her daily life. But as soon as she realized the power of a set place, her chair yoga session became a serene oasis for rest and renewal.

We'll look at the craft of setting up your room for chair yoga in this chapter. We'll walk you through each step, from organizing your space to boosting the ambience, to make sure your practice is enhanced by a setting that promotes your wellbeing and encourages you to completely inhabit the present.

Cleaning Up for Focus

Imagine entering a space that is devoid of clutter, where the air moves easily, and where your mind is at peace. The first step in making a place that supports your chair yoga practice is decluttering. A messy physical space might draw your attention away from the grace of the practice, just as a congested mind can make it difficult to concentrate.

Let's imagine that we are Diane. She is 70 years old and had trouble focusing during her chair yoga sessions. She noticed that the paper piles and other items strewn about the room were competing for her attention with her practice. She started a decluttering quest because she was determined to make a space that encouraged exercise and relaxation.

Diane's story serves as proof of the transforming potential of decluttering. Take the time to evaluate the items around you as you set up your environment. Do they make you feel more at ease and at peace, or do they cause unneeded distractions? You make space for awareness and connection with your practice by getting rid of the clutter.

Increasing Ambience for Serenity

Imagine turning the lights down, lighting a fragrant candle, and opening the door to let a cool air enter. Setting the mood for your chair yoga practice depends heavily on the environment you create. You can encourage a deeper sense of peace in your space by increasing the sensory experience.

Meet Daniel, a 75-year-old dentist who noticed that his clinic lacked ambiance. He chose to include natural elements in his apartment after being inspired by the tranquil settings of healing centers. He strung wind chimes that rustled in the breeze, put potted plants by the window, and put on some background instrumental music.

Daniel's journey demonstrates how the right setting can improve your chair yoga practice. Think about the colors, smells, and sounds that speak to you. The soothing sounds of gentle rain, the scent of lavender, or the warm glow of a Himalayan salt lamp can all help to create an oasis of peace that will assist your practice.

Selecting Comfortable Chairs

Imagine sinking into a comfortable chair that will allow you to concentrate exclusively on the practice that lies ahead. Making your room ready for chair yoga requires careful consideration of your seating options. You are choosing the chair that will support your motions and relaxation, much like a painter chooses the appropriate brush.

Consider Sarah, who began practicing chair yoga on a dining room chair that wasn't quite the right fit for her. She frequently found that the soreness kept her from completely participating in the positions. But after making the purchase of a comfortable and supportive chair, her practice changed. She was now free to move and stretch without being constrained by pain.

Your seating preference is important. Find a robust chair that has a straight back and armrests that you may rest your hands on comfortably. The additional comfort of a padded seat is appreciated. You're building a foundation that enables you to fully immerse yourself in the practice by putting your comfort first.

Setting Up Important Props

Think about having a blanket nearby for times when you need additional comfort or a cushion to raise your seated posture for the best alignment. The correct props can improve your comfort and enable you to completely engage in each posture, elevating your chair yoga practice.

Meet Michael, a 68-year-old who learned the use of supports while participating in chair yoga. As he performed the positions, he found that a cushion may give his spine the ideal amount of lift. Additionally, he discovered that utilizing a strap made it simple for him to deepen his stretches.

Michael's experience emphasizes how crucial it is to set up your environment with the necessary accessories. Think about keeping a yoga strap, a blanket, and a cushion handy. These straightforward tools can significantly improve your practice by enabling you to modify poses to meet your own needs and achieve a deeper state of relaxation.

Putting up a Personal Altar of Inspiration
Imagine a little shrine that is filled with sentimental objects, such as a favorite memento or a statement that makes you smile. Your chair yoga practice will be inspired and more

purposeful if you make a personal altar in your area.

Meet Emma, a 72-year-old who turned to chair yoga for comfort after losing her marriage. She arranged a candle, a framed picture of her marriage, and a tiny container of flowers on an adjacent table to form a modest altar. This altar became a comfort to her, serving as a constant reminder to enter each session with appreciation and a sense of community.

Your personal altar can reflect your beliefs, goals, and the people who make your life enjoyable. It serves as a visual reminder of your practice's aim. Consider the items that are important to you as you settle into your home and organize them in a way that feels right to you.

Opening Your Space to the Sacred

To invite the divine into your life is to create a space that supports your chair yoga practice. Your prepared room becomes a haven of wellbeing and self-care, just like an artist's studio does. The experiences of Laura, Diane, Daniel, Sarah, Michael, and Emma show what a positive difference a well-organized setting can make to your chair yoga practice.

As you begin your trip, take the time to tidy, improve the atmosphere, select comfortable seats, set up necessary props, and build a private altar. Your surroundings serve as a canvas for movement and mindfulness, an extension of your practice. You are creating the foundation for a practice that nurtures your body, mind, and spirit with each attentive detail you include. Let's start by learning the art of setting up your holy place so that each session is a journey toward self-realization and renewal.

Choosing the Right Clothing and Equipment

Imagine entering a world where ease of movement and comfort are one. Every stretch, pose, and breath you take is supported by your clothing, which is an extension of your practice. Choosing appropriate clothing for your chair yoga practice boosts your comfort and enables you to completely enjoy the trip ahead, much as an athlete dons the right gear before a game.

Meet Emma, a 68-year-old who enthusiastically began practicing chair yoga but was unsure of what to wear. She attempted to practice in her regular attire but found that it limited her motions and diminished her enjoyment. But as she came to understand the power of appropriate dress, her practice grew into a place of freedom and self-expression.

We'll go into the art of choosing appropriate chair yoga apparel and gear in this section. We'll walk you through each step, making sure your practice is enhanced by a setting that celebrates your body's strengths and motivates you to discover its potential, from comfortable attire to the support of suitable footwear.

Selecting Cozy and Breathable Clothes
Imagine wearing clothing that is soft, breathable, and receptive to your movements—almost like a second skin. Your experience of chair yoga is greatly influenced by the clothes you choose to wear. Your clothing should provide you the

freedom to move and stretch easily, just like a dancer's outfit facilitates fluid movement.

Consider John, a 75-year-old who began practicing chair yoga while wearing his everyday t-shirt and pants. He quickly understood that his clothing's tight fit was preventing him from fully committing to the positions. He started using loose-fitting slacks and a breathable shirt after being inspired by another practitioner, which allowed him to move freely and fully commit to the practice.

John's experience emphasizes the need of wearing loose-fitting, breathable clothing. Look for clothing with a complete range of motion that is composed of lightweight, elastic materials. Comfort should come first, so make sure your attire gives you the freedom to experiment with each pose with ease and confidence.

Choosing Supportive Shoes

Consider moving through the poses while wearing shoes that hug your feet and offer stability and support. The appropriate footwear can improve your entire experience and sense of balance even if chair yoga is mostly a seated practice.

Meet Sarah, a 70-year-old who started out performing chair yoga in her everyday pajamas. Although they were cozy, she discovered that they lacked the grip and stability required for several standing poses. She bought a pair of sturdy, non-slip sneakers when she started incorporating standing and balancing chair yoga routines. With this minor adjustment, she was able to expand the scope of her profession without risking her safety.

Sarah's experience highlights the importance of wearing supportive shoes. Search for footwear with an arch support, padding, and a non-slip sole. Even though chair yoga is generally done while sitting down, wearing the proper shoes will guarantee that you are ready for any standing or balancing motions.

Wearing only minimal jewelry as decoration

Imagine being able to practice yoga without feeling restricted by a lot of jewelry. When wearing less jewelry when practicing chair yoga is a sensible choice that assures your comfort and safety, accessories can be a way to display one's personality.

Consider Michael, a 68-year-old who was used to doing chair yoga while wearing his watch, rings, and bracelets. He soon noticed that these objects were making him uncomfortable and making it difficult for him to completely engage in the positions. He felt a new sense of freedom and ease by removing his jewelry for the duration of his practice.

The value of wearing little jewelry is illustrated through Michael's experience. Consider putting away things that can restrict your motions or make you uncomfortable as you get ready for practice. By giving oneself the freedom to practice without interruption, you're fostering an atmosphere where movement and mindfulness take the lead.

Utilizing Layers to Manage Temperature

Imagine yourself in a place where you are comfortable—not too hot or cold—where you can concentrate entirely on your practice without being disturbed by outside influences. By dressing in layers, you can adjust to shifting temperatures and make sure that you're comfortable the entire time.

Let's assume Mark's position. He's a 70-year-old man who started out doing chair yoga while only wearing one layer of clothing. But as he changed positions and movements, he observed that his body temperature changed. He occasionally felt too warm and other times he was chilled. He discovered that he could easily alter his clothing to suit his body's needs by adding layers to it.

The importance of layers in your chair yoga outfit is highlighted by Mark's experience. Pick up outfits that let you add or remove layers as necessary. This flexibility makes sure that you can concentrate on your practice without being distracted by changes in temperature.

Prioritizing ease of use and expression

In addition to being functional, what you wear gives you a chance to express yourself. The way you dress can increase your connection to your profession and represent your personality, just as an artist's palette shows their own style.

Imagine Jane, a 65-year-old who made the decision to dress in brilliant colors and patterns that made her happy for her chair yoga practice. She discovered that dressing in ways that reflected her sense of self made her feel better and provided a positive element to her practice. Her outfit became a symbol of her dedication to self-care and discovery each time she entered her practice area.

Jane's experience emphasizes the value of putting comfort first while still adding your own flair to your wardrobe. Dress in a way that gives you a sense of empowerment, assurance, and connection to your practice. Let your wardrobe be a representation of the adventure you're about to take, whether it's a favorite color, a meaningful pattern, or just clothing that feels like an extension of yourself.

Enhancing Your Practice With Proper Clothes and Equipment

Your wardrobe and tools raise your chair yoga practice, much as a dancer's costume might improve their performance. The experiences of Emma, John, Sarah, Michael, Mark, and Jane show the transformational effects that appropriate clothes and equipment may have on your profession.

Consider these factors as you get ready for your chair yoga sessions: dress in loose-fitting, breathable clothing; choose supportive footwear; wear little jewelry; embrace layers for temperature regulation; and give equal weight to comfort and individuality. You may foster a space where movement and mindfulness are seamlessly interwoven into one experience by **Approaching your practice with intention and consideration.**

In addition to being practical considerations, your clothing and equipment serve as an invitation to appreciate your body, embrace your practice, and set out on a path to wellbeing. Let's improve your chair yoga experience by mastering the art of appropriate clothing and gear, making each session a celebration of movement, comfort, and self-expression.

Chapter 3

Fundamentals of Chair Yoga

Breathing Techniques for Relaxation

Think of a soft breeze that whispers through the trees, bringing peace and tranquility to the atmosphere. Your breath has the ability to bring peace and presence, just as nature's rhythm does. Here, the act of inhaling and exhaling becomes a doorway to inner serenity. This is the world of chair yoga breathing practices.

Meet Emily, a 70-year-old who once thought breathing was a natural function that didn't involve any deliberate effort. But as she got more into chair yoga, she realized that breathing could be a transforming technique for awareness and relaxation. Her road to breathing technique mastery unlocked doors to a peaceful world she had never envisioned.

We'll explore the skill of chair yoga breathing methods in this chapter. We'll look at a variety of techniques, like deep belly breathing and guided relaxation, to help you unlock the potential of your breath and incorporate relaxation into every aspect of your practice and life.

Understanding the Benefits of Deep Breathing

Think about pausing to focus on your breath and seeing how it flows in and out like the tides of the ocean. Deep belly breathing is a key chair yoga practice that uses the breath's natural rhythm to promote attention and relaxation.

Take Robert for example, a 68-year-old who frequently found himself entangled in the maelstrom of daily worries. He first learned how to do deep belly breathing in a chair yoga lesson. He followed the instructor's instructions to take slow, deep breaths that stretched his tummy with each inhalation as he relaxed comfortably in his chair. Robert was surprised by the overwhelming sense of serenity that came over him right away.

Robert's experience serves as an example of the effectiveness of deep belly breathing in reducing stress and calming the nervous system. You can cause the body to relax by deliberately guiding your breath into your abdomen. You're gently pushing stress aside with each breath and expiration to make room for peace to enter.

Guided Relaxation: A Trip Inside

Imagine being led through a peaceful setting, full peace, the feel of warm sun on your skin, and the sound of soft waves. A chair yoga method called guided relaxation transports you mentally to a serene location.

Meet Sarah, a 72-year-old who frequently had anxiety and insomnia. She first encountered guided relaxation in her chair yoga session. Sarah felt the strain leave her body as the instructor's calming voice guided her through an image of a tranquil garden. She felt physically calmed by the exercise, and it also provided a break from the worries that frequently kept her up at night.

Sarah's experience serves to highlight the significant benefits of guided relaxation. You may create a calm sanctuary inside by utilizing your imagination and concentration. You can use guided relaxation as a strategy to reduce stress and find comfort in quiet moments even after you stop practicing.

The practice of conscious breathing

Take a moment to picture yourself strolling through a forest, each step deliberate and mindful of your surroundings. By focusing your attention on the pattern of your breath, mindful breathing is a chair yoga technique that invites you to be fully present with each inhalation and expiration.

Take Michael, a 65-year-old who frequently experienced disorientation and overwhelm due to the demands of modern life. He learned the technique of attentive breathing during his chair yoga lessons. He concentrated on the sensation of his breath entering and exiting his body as he sat in his chair. He had a sense of balance and presence with each breath cycle that escaped him for years.

Michael's experience exemplifies the value of mindful breathing in fostering the capacity for the moment. You gently nudge distractions aside and embrace the present moment by focusing on your breath. An anchor that holds you in the here and now, attentive breathing enables you to experience each moment with clarity and mindfulness.

The Ujjayi Breathing Symphony

Imagine the rhythmic, calming melody of ocean waves crashing across the coast, lulling you into a state of tranquility. Ujjayi breathing, sometimes known as "ocean breath," is a chair yoga practice in which you breathe while slightly tightening the back of your throat to produce a mellow, ocean-like sound.

You should get to know Diane, a 75-year-old woman who frequently battled anxiety that seemed to swell like ocean waves. She was introduced to ujjayi breathing by her chair yoga instructor as a way to control her worried thoughts. As she continued to use this approach, she discovered that the comforting sound of her breath was similar to the sound of waves lapping against the coast.

Diane's experience demonstrates how ujjayi breathing may be comforting. You can activate the body's relaxation response and promote inner tranquility by making a soothing sound as you breathe. You can connect with your breath and find comfort in its rhythm by practicing ujjayi breathing, which turns into a tune that helps you get through your practice.

Harmonizing the breath with the body
A symphony of relaxation and mindfulness is created by synchronizing your body and breath with chair yoga breathing methods. The

experiences of Emily, Robert, Sarah, Michael, and Diane demonstrate how these techniques for calming the mind, calming the nerve system, and promoting awareness of the present moment.

You are building a toolkit of relaxation techniques that you may incorporate into your daily life as you practice guided relaxation, mindful breathing, deep belly breathing, and ujjayi breathing. You can handle tension, worry, and restlessness with the help of these approaches. Every inhale and expiration becomes a chance to find peace within, building a path to a place of inner tranquility and wellbeing.

So let's start the path of learning breathing exercises from chair yoga to perfect relaxation.

You're unlocking the entrance to a calm haven with each breath you take—a place where the seemingly insignificant act of breathing takes on a profound and enlightening practice.

Mind-Body Connection

Imagine dancing in a way where each step is dictated by your ideas and each thought is supported by each action. The connected mind and body form a delicate dance that affects your experiences and general wellbeing; they are not two distinct things. Welcome to the world of chair yoga's exploration of the mind-body link, which aims to close the gap between your inner self and your physical self.

Introducing David, a 60-year-old who formerly thought that his body and mind functioned independently. He soon learned that the mind-body link was a route to overall healing, though, as he dug further into his chair yoga practice. He started to comprehend the deep effect of this relationship on his general sense of well-being through mindfulness and purposeful movement.

We'll explore the art of the mind-body connection in chair yoga in this chapter. We'll examine the transforming potential of matching your thoughts with your movements, generating a profound sense of harmony between your inner world and physical body, from developing self-awareness to engaging in mindfulness.

Self-Awareness Development Through Movement

Think about having a keen awareness of your body's sensations and reactions as you go about your daily activities. Chair yoga presents a special chance to develop self-awareness by encouraging you to pay attention to each stretch, movement, and breath.

Take Susan, a 65-year-old woman who started off by treating chair yoga like a set of exercises. She saw a deeper connection building though as she started to pay attention to the minute changes in her body that occurred with each stance. She was aware of the feelings that arose with each movement, the slight stretch in her muscles, and the rise and fall of her breath. She was able to interact with her practice on a completely new level as a result of her newly acquired awareness.

Susan's experience demonstrates the value of developing self-awareness through exercise. Pay close attention to how your body responds to each posture as you perform chair yoga. Keep an eye out for the points of tension, the feelings of release, and the times of ease. By bridging the gap between your body and mind, this mindful awareness technique fosters a deeper understanding of who you are.

Opening the Door to a Journey of Mindful Movement

Think of your chair yoga practice as a moving meditation that anchors you in the here and now, as you go through it with a sense of presence and intention. Integrating your thoughts and actions is the art of mindful movement, which transforms your routine into a journey of mindfulness and self-awareness.

Meet Anna, a 72-year-old chair yoga practitioner who frequently experienced mind wandering. Everything changed when she started to approach her practice mindfully, though. She felt her breath match with her motions, felt her chest gently rise and fall, and observed how her body reacted to each stretch. Her practice changed into a sort of meditation in action as a result of her deliberate focus.

Anna's story serves as an example of how mindful movement can be transformational. Invite your focus to remain with each movement and each breath as you perform chair yoga. Allow your ideas to match your actions, building a link between your inner world and your physical sensations. This exercise not only improves your chair yoga experience, but it also carries over into your daily life and cultivates mindfulness and presence.

Through breathing and movement, you may create harmony.

Imagine creating a dance where each inhalation and exhalation is choreographed with a specific goal. When you breathe in time with your movements, generating a continuous flow of energy and awareness, you can really feel the mind-body connection in chair yoga.

Take James, a 68-year-old who originally found it difficult to control his breath and motions while doing chair yoga. He observed a sense of togetherness forming as he persisted and concentrated on matching his inhales and exhales with each stance. The breath served as a guide, directing him into each action and assisting him in making smooth transitions.

James's experience demonstrates the potency of bringing harmony to movement and breath. Try synchronizing your breath with each pose as you perform chair yoga. Breathe in to expand and out to release. Your physical movements are improved by this synchronization, which also strengthens your mind-body bond and gives you a feeling of flow and presence.

Promoting mindfulness in each posture
Imagine being completely present in every moment, with your thoughts and actions working in one. The chair yoga practice invites you to be fully involved with each position and movement, cultivating a state of enhanced

awareness and presence. Mindfulness is the cornerstone of the mind-body connection.

Meet Karen, a 70-year-old woman whose worries and other distractions frequently set her thoughts spinning. She learned the value of mindfulness in establishing a solid foundation for her thoughts and emotions through her chair yoga practice. She concentrated on the physical sensations, the rise and fall of her breath, and how her body responded to each stance as she practiced it. She was able to calm down and let go of the mental chatter thanks to her deliberate focus.

Karen's story serves as an excellent example of the deep benefits of mindfulness in chair yoga. Invite your attention to focus on the present moment as you perform each pose. Take note of the specifics of each motion, your physical sensations, and the consistency of your breathing. By encouraging mindfulness, you're building a connection between your mind and body, resulting in a profound sense of presence and wellbeing.

The dance that unites the body and mind.
In chair yoga, the mind-body connection is like a dance—a harmonic interplay of thoughts and motions that promotes equilibrium and well-being. The experiences of David, Susan, Anna, James, and Karen demonstrate the transformational potential of thinking in harmony with your physical self.

You are building a holy bridge that connects your inner world with your physical body as you practice self-awareness, mindful movement, breath-synchronized movement, and mindfulness in each pose. In your chair yoga practice and in your life in general, this bridge turns into a route to present, self-discovery, and a deeper feeling of balance.

In order to dance through life with elegance, mindfulness, and a profound sense of well-being, let's embrace the art of the mind-body connection in chair yoga—a journey that transcends the lines between thought and action.

Chapter 4

Seated Poses for Flexibility

Gentle Stretches for Every Body

Think of your body like a river, versatile, and able to flow across different environments. You are invited to practice chair yoga to discover your body's flexibility, connect with its natural movements, and enjoy the pleasure of gentle stretches that respect your individual capacities. Your body can go through stretches that provide a sensation of freedom and vitality, much as a river winds between hills and valleys.

Meet Sarah, a 75-year-old woman who thought that growing older had made her body less flexible. She discovered a world of gentle stretches through her chair yoga practice, though, and was able to rediscover the possibilities of her body. She discovered through diligent effort and patient experimentation that flexibility is about moving comfortably and easily, nourishing her body's wellbeing, rather than just achieving extreme poses.

We'll set off on a journey of gentle chair yoga stretches for every body in this chapter. We'll look at a variety of stretches that highlight your body's special qualities and lead you to a state of increased flexibility and relaxation, from neck and shoulder releases to seated spinal twists.

Stretching the Shoulders and Neck Can Help You Feel Better

Imagine the tension in your neck and shoulders dissipating in a cascade of releases that leaves you feeling light and refreshed. Chair yoga's neck and shoulder stretches are like a gentle massage for these frequently stiff areas, giving you a feeling of comfort and relaxation.

Take Michael, a 68-year-old who frequently experienced discomfort in his neck and shoulders as a result of spending numerous hours at a computer. He felt a new sensation of freedom as he added neck and shoulder stretches to his chair yoga regimen. Even small movements like shifting his shoulders or tilting his head to one side could provide brief moments of respite.

Michael's experience highlights the effectiveness of chair yoga's neck and shoulder stretches. Take breaks throughout the day to perform these stretches. Roll your shoulders forward and backward, gently tilt your head from side to side, and let your neck relax any tension that has built up. These stretches provide a brief opportunity for self-care that can significantly improve your comfort and wellbeing.

Twists while seated can help to maintain spinal health.

Think of your spine as a flexible vine that can bend and twirl gracefully, supporting the motions of your body. Chair yoga's seated spinal twists offer moderate rotation that improves flexibility and promotes a sensation of vigor,

76

which is a way to care for the health of your spine.

Meet Emily, a 70-year-old who frequently experienced back tightness as a result of a sedentary lifestyle. She gained an appreciation for seated spinal twists through her chair yoga practice. She gradually turned her torso while sitting and felt a wonderful relaxation in her back. She pictured her spine getting more flexible with each twist, like a river passing through various vistas.

Emily's story demonstrates the seated spinal twists' transforming potential. As you perform these twists, visualize the movement of each vertebra. Respecting your body's range of motion requires careful action. These stretches give you a chance to improve the health of your spine and experience the joy of movement.

Stretching the Chest to Open the Heart

Think of your heart as a warm, glowing sun that emitted light and warmth. Chair yoga's chest stretches encourage you to open your heart, letting go of tension and experiencing a feeling of expansion and well-being.

Take David, a 60-year-old man who frequently experienced tension in his chest as a result of bad posture. He found comfort in chest stretches that prompted him to sit up straight and widen his heart during his chair yoga sessions. The feeling of freedom he experienced when he opened his arms wide and drew his shoulder blades together was similar to the sensation of sunlight penetrating clouds.

David's experience demonstrates how chest stretches may change your life. By interlacing your fingers behind your back and gradually elevating your arms, letting your chest expand, you can incorporate these stretches into your practice. Visualize your heart expanding and your breath being unrestricted. These stretches invite you to embrace openness and let go of stress, providing a moment of regeneration.

Stretching the Hips While Seated Can Relieve Pain

Think of your hips as the structural center of your body, providing stability and support. In chair yoga, seated hip stretches are a great technique to relax your hips, loosen up, and develop a groundedness.

Meet Karen, a 70-year-old who frequently felt pain in her hips from spending a lot of time sitting down. She discovered sitting hip stretches during her chair yoga practice, allowing her to experiment with soft motions that nourished her hip joints. She envisioned her hips achieving harmony and balance as she slowly rocked from side to side, much like a river finding its course.

Karen's experience emphasizes how crucial seated hip stretches are. By slowly moving your hips from side to side or bringing one leg at a time closer to your chest, you can include these stretches into your practice. Consider gentle exercises that feel soothing and liberating for your hips. These stretches promote communication to strengthen the structure of your body and encourage stability.

Gentle Stretches while Flowing with Freedom

Stretching gently is a celebration of your body's adaptability and toughness. The experiences of Sarah, Michael, Emily, David, and Karen show the transformational impact of accepting the potential of your body via simple stretches.

You may invite a feeling of freedom and vigor into your body by relaxing your neck and shoulders, promoting spinal health with sat twists, opening your heart with chest stretches, and soothing your hips with seated hip stretches. Each stretch serves as a gateway to increased flexibility, calmness, and a closer relationship with your body's intrinsic intelligence.

In order to acknowledge your body's individual potential, promote wellbeing, and enable you to move through life with ease and grace, let's embrace the art of gentle stretches for every body in chair yoga.

Enhancing Joint Mobility

Think of your joints as the hinges that enable graceful, effortless movement of your body. By improving joint mobility, chair yoga enables you to appreciate the flexibility of your body's motions. This discovery transcends age-related limits and fosters a sense of vitality and well-being. The gentle practice of chair yoga can influence your body's movement, much like a river's flow is guided by its path.

Meet Alex, a 72-year-old who felt that as he got older, his joints were getting stiffer and less supple. However, he realized that joint mobility was more than just a theoretical potential through his chair yoga practice; it was a voyage of empowerment and self-discovery. He discovered that his joints may regain their flexibility and contribute to a life of comfort and movement with time and effort.

We'll set out on a journey in this chapter to improve joint mobility using chair yoga. We'll look at a variety of exercises that celebrate the potential of your joints, allowing you to move through life with a fresh sense of freedom and ease. These range from modest wrist and ankle movements to full-body circles.

How to Take Care of Your Wrists and Ankles
Consider your wrists and ankles as the complex systems that enable your hands and feet to move about the outside world. Chair yoga gives a means to take care of these important joints by enhancing their mobility and preventing stiffness with gentle exercises.

Consider Lisa, a 65-year-old who, as a result of her sedentary lifestyle, frequently experienced pain in her wrists and ankles. She experienced relaxation and renewal when she added wrist and ankle exercises to her chair yoga routine. She was able to interact with her body's potential for movement and flexibility by doing something as easy as circling her wrists or flexing her ankles.

Lisa's story emphasizes how crucial it is to take good care of your wrists and ankles. Take breaks throughout the day to perform these exercises. Pay attention to the feelings in your ankles and wrists as you slowly circle them. These movements provide a brief opportunity for self-care that can reduce stiffness and enhance joint health.

Activating the Hips and Shoulders

Think of your shoulders and hips as the joints that link your movements with your upper and lower bodies. Through gentle movements that promote mobility and range of motion, chair yoga offers a platform for revitalizing these crucial joints.

Meet Daniel, a 75-year-old man with a sedentary lifestyle who frequently had tightness and stiffness in his shoulders and hips. He discovered movements that allowed him to carefully and intentionally examine these areas through his chair yoga practice. He had a newfound sense of mobility and flexibility that went beyond his practice, from seated shoulder rolls to hip circles.

The importance of energizing the shoulders and hips is highlighted by Daniel's experience. By gently rotating your hips while seated or rolling your shoulders forward and backward, you can incorporate these exercises into your practice. These exercises provide a feeling of vibrancy and release while promoting joint mobility.

Maintaining Spinal Flexibility

Think of your spine as a supple reed that can flow with the wind and conform to the curves of your movements. Through moderate twists and bends, chair yoga techniques promote spinal flexibility, giving your spine a sense of freedom and fluidity.

Take Laura, a 62-year-old who frequently noticed that her sedentary employment was causing her spine to become rigid and immovable. She discovered the delight of spine flexibility exercises through her chair yoga practice. She felt her spine reacting with a fresh suppleness as she slowly twisted her torso and leaned side to side. She visualized her spine embracing its innate capacity for adaptation and movement with each motion.

Laura's story demonstrates the positive effects of promoting spine flexibility. Leaning from side to side while gently twisting your torso can help you incorporate these movements into your practice. Consider your spine as a river running across many landscapes, finding its rhythm and flexibility. These exercises provide you a chance to develop your spine's sense of freedom and movement.

Exercises for Joint Mobility Help You Flow Easily

A celebration of your body's flexibility and resiliency is increased joint mobility. The experiences of Alex, Lisa, Daniel, and Laura show how embracing joint mobility in chair yoga has the power to alter.

You are embarking on a path that encourages comfort, flexibility, and vitality as you exercise your joints and take care of your wrists and ankles, shoulders, and hips. Your body will become more flexible and receptive with each movement, enabling you to navigate through life with grace and ease.

Let's thus begin our adventure into the art of improving joint mobility with chair yoga—a trip that respects your body's capacity for movement, promotes wellbeing, and invites you to flow through life with ease and vibrancy.

Chapter 5

Strengthening Your Core and Balance

Building Core Stability

Think of your core as the strong base that underpins each movement you make—a source of strength that stabilizes your frame and motivates your behavior. You are invited to explore the potential of developing core stability through chair yoga—a journey that goes beyond the obvious and develops a profound sense of strength and balance. Your core may anchor you in a world of movement and well-being, much to how a tree's roots give it solidity in the wind.

Meet Emily, a 68-year-old who thought that core strength was something that only athletes and fitness fanatics cared about. However, she became aware of the transforming power of developing core stability through her chair yoga practice. She discovered that developing core strength was about developing a sense of inner strength and resilience rather than achieving extreme poses via persistent practice and attentive participation.

We'll go into the process of developing core stability in chair yoga in this chapter. We'll look at a variety of exercises that highlight the potential for strength, balance, and wellbeing in your body, from easy seated twists to focused core activation.

Twists while seated: Activating Core Engagement

Think of your inner strength as a spiraling force, a coiled spring of energy that responds to your motions with elegance and stability. Chair yoga's seated twists provide a means to activate and fortify your core muscles, fostering a sense of balance and fortitude.

Take Michael, a 70-year-old who frequently experienced weakness in his core as a result of a sedentary lifestyle. He enjoyed seated twists that allowed him to purposefully engage his core during his chair yoga practice. His core muscles began to awaken as he gently twisted from side to side, giving him a sense of strength and vigor.

Michael's experience demonstrates the healing power of chair yoga's seated twists. Sit tall and gradually rotate your torso to incorporate these twists into your routine. Think of your core muscles waking up and contracting with each motion. Along with strengthening the core, these twists also promote alignment and balance.

Finding Your Center: Targeted Core Engagement

Think of your core as a compass—an internal compass that regulates your posture and movements. Chair yoga offers a platform for focused core engagement exercises that aid in centering you, building a solid base for your practice and daily life.

Meet Sarah, a 75-year-old who frequently experienced back pain and bad posture. She found specific core engagement exercises that enabled her to connect with her deep core muscles through her chair yoga practice. She felt a sense of solidity emanating from her center as she tightened her abdominal muscles and slowly pulled them inside. She visualized her core strengthening with each engagement, supporting the motions of her body.

The necessity of targeted core activation in chair yoga is highlighted by Sarah's experience. Sit comfortably while performing these exercises by gently contracting your abdominal muscles. Think of pulling them upward and within, giving them a sense of security. These interactions provide an opportunity to develop inner strength and a solid foundation.

A Symphony of Strength: Breathing and the Core

With each inhale and exhalation, picture your breath as the rhythm that synchronizes with the motions of your core, creating a dance of strength and balance. Chair yoga encourages a symphony of stability and vibrancy by inviting you to investigate the relationship between breathing and core engagement.

Take John, a 68-year-old who frequently thought his core muscles were not attached to him. He learned the value of breathing as a tool to activate and strengthen his core through his chair yoga practice. He visualized his breath expanding his belly and working his abs as he inhaled. He experienced a slight constriction with each breath that gave him a sense of steadiness and power.

John's experience exemplifies the ability of breathing and core connection in chair yoga to transform. Try synchronizing your breath with your core contraction as you get more practice. Exhale to release after inhaling to expand and engage. Your core's strength and stability are improved by this rhythmic connection, which promotes a strong sensation of equilibrium and wellbeing.

Core strength in action with balancing poses
Think of your core as an anchor, a center of gravity that enables you to maintain equilibrium

and stability in a world that is constantly in motion. Chair yoga's balancing postures give you a chance to use your core strength, which promotes balance and self-assurance.

Introducing Lisa, a 60-year-old who frequently felt clumsy and uncertain in her movements. She learned balancing poses that helped her to use her core muscles and gain equilibrium through her chair yoga practice. She felt her core responding with strength and support as she lifted one foot off the ground or spread her arms outward. She visualized her core supporting her body and giving her a newfound sense of stability with each balancing stance.

Lisa's experience highlights the beneficial qualities of chair yoga's balance postures. By experimenting with elevating one foot or extending your arms while seated, you can include these positions into your practice. Imagine your core muscles holding you in a stable position as you contract them. These positions not only increase core strength but also balance and self-assurance.

The fortress within which core stability resides.

Exploring inner strength and resilience is a part of creating core stability. The experiences of Emily, Michael, Sarah, John, and Lisa demonstrate the transforming power of developing core stability in chair yoga.

You're building a solid foundation from the inside out as you practice seated twists, focus on core engagement, link breathing and core, and appreciate balancing poses. Your core develops into a source of stability and strength that supports your posture, movements, and general well-being. Every workout becomes a way to develop a stronger feeling of equilibrium and inner toughness.

So let's start the adventure of developing core stability in chair yoga, a trip that celebrates the strength and balancing potential of your body and gives you the tools to face life's challenges with fortitude and assurance.

Improving Balance and Coordination

Think of your body as a dancer's: fluid, poised, and capable of graceful, accurate movement. Chair yoga enables you to engage in a journey that goes beyond physical motions and connects with your inner rhythms—a stage of balance and coordination. Your body can be guided by the gentle practice of chair yoga, just as a dancer's motions are influenced by music.

Meet Maria, a 70-year-old who thought she had lost her ability to balance and coordinate in her youth. She was nonetheless introduced to a world where these traits might be fostered and enhanced at any age through her chair yoga practice. She discovered that balance and coordination were not far-off ideals, but rather attainable goals that improved her general well-being through focused attention and attentive actions.

We'll explore the process of developing balance and coordination with chair yoga in this chapter. We'll examine a range of exercises that honor your body's capacity for harmony, elegance, and movement, from straightforward weight shifts to dynamic flowing sequences.

Weight Shifts While Seated: Locating Your Center

Consider your body as a finely tuned balance, a series of weight changes that enable you to move steadily and intentionally. Chair yoga's seated weight transfers provide a gradual introduction to bettering balance and coordination and lay the groundwork for more difficult postures.

Take Alex, a 65-year-old man who frequently felt clumsy and uncertain in his actions. He learned about the transformational power of seated weight changes through his chair yoga practice. While sitting, he felt connected to his body's center of gravity by adjusting his weight from side to side or forward and backward. He visualized his body regaining equilibrium and alignment with each shift.

The importance of chair yoga's seated weight transfers is shown by Alex's experience. Try exploring with soft motions while sitting and incorporating these exercises into your practice. As you change your weight, visualize your body's center of gravity to develop awareness and balance. These changes provide you more space to connect with your body's natural rhythms while also enhancing your coordination.

Dynamic Flowing Sequences: A Graceful Movement

Think of your body as a river that can flow through a variety of terrain with ease, adaptation, and fluidity. Chair yoga's dynamic, flowing sequences offer the chance to enhance balance and coordination through a series of interconnected motions that honor your body's natural ability to flow and be graceful.

Meet Daniel, a sedentary 72-year-old who frequently felt distant from his body's actions. He learned dynamic flowing sequences that enabled him to investigate movement in a fresh way through his chair yoga practice. He felt his body responding with a novel sense of coordination as he performed modest twists and stretches, raised his arms aloft, and leaned side to side. He visualized his body evolving into a graceful, purposeful river of movement with each flowing cycle.

Daniel's experience demonstrates the transforming power of chair yoga's dynamic, flowing sequences. Link simple motions together fluidly to create these sequences in your practice. Visualize your body flowing from one pose to the next with elegance and intention. These movements not only help with coordination but also promote inner peace and flow.

Poses on One Leg: Embracing Balance

Think of your body as a tree: firmly planted, sturdy, and able to sway with the wind without losing its base. In chair yoga, one-legged postures provide a chance to enhance balance and coordination by concentrating on the power and steadiness of a single leg, fostering a sense of rootedness and poise.

Take Mia, a 68-year-old woman who frequently felt unsteady and unsure when standing on one leg. She became aware of the one-legged poses' capacity for transformation through her chair yoga practice. She felt a sense of connection with the natural steadiness of her body as she raised one foot off the ground and regained her balance. She pictured herself planted like a tree in each stance, embracing strength and balance.

The value of one-legged poses in chair yoga is emphasized by Mia's experience. Lift one foot off the ground while seated while performing these poses, or grasp onto the back of a chair for support. Think of your body gaining equilibrium and solidity, similar to a tree standing tall. These postures help you feel grounded and confident while also enhancing your balance.

The heartbeat of coordination and balance is mindfulness.

You can move with intention and precision by visualizing your awareness as a spotlight that illuminates your body's motions. Chair yoga, a form of exercise that encourages a strong connection between your mind and body, places a strong emphasis on mindful awareness as a way to improve balance and coordination.

Take Sarah, a 75-year-old woman who frequently felt detached from her body's motions. She learned the value of attentive awareness in enhancing her balance and coordination through chair yoga practice. She felt her body responding with a greater feeling of coordination and grace as she concentrated her attention on each movement, each breath, and each experience. She visualized herself dancing through life with elegance and awareness, making each attentive movement with intention and presence.

The transformational potential of focused awareness in chair yoga is demonstrated by

Sarah's experience. Practice each movement while paying close attention to it. Visualize your awareness controlling your physical movements, enabling you to move with purpose and accuracy. Along with enhancing your coordination, this exercise promotes a strong bond between your mind and body.

The harmony of equilibrium and coordination

Harmony, elegance, and presence are explored in the process of improving balance and coordination. The experiences of Maria, Alex, Daniel, Mia, and Sarah highlight the transforming potential of encouraging balance and coordination in chair yoga.

You're stepping into a realm of movement that honors your body's capacity for grace and balance as you practice sitting weight transfers, investigate dynamic flowing sequences, accept one-legged postures, and develop mindful awareness. Each exercise serves as a stepping stone toward better coordination, a closer relationship with your body, and a sense of fluid movement.

Let's start a chair yoga adventure to improve balance and coordination. This trip will awaken the inner dancer, promote wellbeing, and challenge you to move through life with grace, poise, and attentive awareness.

Chapter 6

Cardiovascular Chair Exercises

Improving Heart Health

Imagine your heart as a tireless conductor, guiding you through each moment as it rhythmically beats, pumping life into your body. By improving heart health, chair yoga invites you to take care of your lifeline—a journey that goes beyond simple physical activity and embraces the harmony between your heart and well-being. Chair yoga is a moderate exercise that can be used to support the health of your heart, much like a conductor does for an orchestra.

A 68-year-old man named Robert thought his heart health was a faraway problem that he didn't need to address. However, he discovered via his chair yoga practice that improving heart health was a journey of empowerment and self-care. He discovered that heart health was not just about cardiovascular fitness, but also about developing a relationship with his heart that boosted his general vitality through attentive movements and focused breathing.

We'll go into the process of improving heart health in chair yoga in this chapter. We'll look at a variety of activities that celebrate the health of your heart and inspire a feeling of harmony and vigor, ranging from light cardiovascular workouts to heart-centered mindfulness.

Exercises for Your Heart's Fitness: Cardiovascular

Think of your heart as a robust muscle that flourishes when it is active and engaged. Through easy cardiovascular activities that encourage circulation, improve your cardiovascular system, and add to a feeling of vigor, chair yoga offers a means to nurture the health of your heart.

Take Emily, a 70-year-old who frequently experienced heart palpitations as a result of stress and a sedentary lifestyle. She learned about the transformational power of cardiovascular activity through her chair yoga practice. She felt her heart responding with a sensation of awakening as she performed rhythmic foot tapping, soft jumping jacks, and seated marching. She envisioned her heart finding its beat with each motion, much like a tune in a song.

The importance of cardiovascular workouts in chair yoga is brought home by Emily's experience. Gently moving while seated will raise your heart rate, so incorporate these exercises into your practice. As you move, visualize your heart pumping to increase circulation and vigor. These exercises not only improve the health of your heart, but they also provide you a chance to tune into the rhythms of your body.

Breath and Heart Connection: A Wellness Symphony

Consider your breath as the song that follows your heartbeat and directs the actions of your body while nourishing your wellbeing. By synchronizing your breath with your heart's rhythm and promoting a wellness symphony, chair yoga's breath and heart connection offers a technique to improve heart health.

Meet Maria, a 65-year-old woman who frequently felt cut off from her physical experiences. She learned the importance of connecting the heart and breath through her chair yoga practice. She experienced alignment and present as she timed her breath with her heartbeat. She imagined her heart establishing a regular beat with each inhale and expiration, as though a soft drumming accompanied her motions.

Maria's experience exemplifies the power of chair yoga's breath and heart connection to transform. Try to time your breathing to the beat of your heart as you practice. Breathe in as your heart beats and out when it relaxes. In addition to promoting the health of your heart, this relationship also promotes inner harmony and wellbeing.

The Inner Pulse: Mindful Heart-Centered Awareness

Consider your awareness as a soft touch that allows you to tune into your heart's rhythms, hear its whispers, and take care of its needs. Through the promotion of a strong connection between your mind and heart, chair yoga offers a practice that improves heart health.

Take John, a 72-year-old man whose anxiousness frequently caused his heart to race. He learned about the transformational potential of attentive heart-centered awareness through his chair yoga practice. He focused on his heart, picturing it as a place of peace and equilibrium. He experienced his heart reacting to his goal with each breath, achieving balance and serenity.

The importance of focused heart-centered awareness in chair yoga is highlighted by John's experience. Practice each action with your heart at the center of your attention. Imagine your awareness nourishing the health of your heart, allowing it to discover its own rhythm. This routine promotes a strong bond between your mind and heart in addition to improving heart health.

Heart-Opening Pose: Promoting Vitality and Love

Think of your heart as a place where compassion, vitality, and wellbeing all come together. Through gentle chest stretching, improved circulation, and a sensation of openness and vibrancy, heart-opening chair yoga poses offer a way to improve heart health.

Meet Laura, a 62-year-old woman who frequently experienced chest discomfort as a result of bad posture. She learned about the heart-opening poses' capacity for transformation through her chair yoga practice. She felt her chest opening and her heart space enlarging when she softly spread her arms wide or interlaced her fingers behind her back. She imagined her heart embracing a sensation of love and vibrancy with each stance.

Laura's experience highlights the value of chair yoga positions that expand the heart. Stretching your arms and chest while seated will help you achieve these poses. Imagine the area of your heart enlarging to give you a feeling of openness and vigor. These positions not only improve heart health but also foster a sense of wellbeing and affection.

The harmony of a strong heart
Exploring harmony, connection, and energy is a key component of improving heart health. The

experiences of Robert, Emily, Maria, John, and Laura show the transforming potential of encouraging heart health in chair yoga.

You can generate a sense of wellbeing that radiates from the inside out by doing cardiovascular exercises, connecting breath and heart, developing attentive heart-centered awareness, and embracing heart-opening positions. Each exercise becomes a step on the route to a heart that is healthier, a closer relationship with your body, and a sense of balance and vigor.

In order to improve heart health, let's practice chair yoga. This journey will celebrate your heart's rhythm, promote wellbeing, and

challenge you to live life with a sense of
connection, love, and vitality.

Low-Impact Cardio for Seniors

Think of your heart as a priceless diamond that has to be treated with the highest respect. Through low-impact cardio, chair yoga inspires you to embrace heart-friendly movement—a path that goes beyond intense exercise and nurtures the health of your heart. Through the peaceful practice of chair yoga, your heart can glitter with life much like a jewel does.

Introducing Grace, a 72-year-old who thought her days of engaging in heart-healthy activity were over. However, she discovered a world of low-impact cardio that was not only doable but also incredibly advantageous through her chair yoga practice. She learned that heart-friendly exercise was a method to respect her body's requirements and contribute to her general well-being through attentive movements and intentional breathing.

This chapter will examine the development of chair yoga as low-impact cardio for seniors. We'll enjoy the power of movement that nourishes your heart and beckons a sense of vigor and joy, from rhythmic breathing exercises to gentle cardiovascular motions.

Exercises for Rhythmic Breathing: Harmonizing Breath and Heart

Think of your breath as a steady rhythm, a kind conductor that directs the pulse of your heart and helps your body move. By synchronizing your breath with your heart and promoting a sense of serenity and wellbeing, chair yoga's rhythmic breathing techniques provide a method to enjoy heart-friendly movement.

Take Robert, a 68-year-old man who frequently experienced tension and anxiety. He learned about the transformational power of rhythmic breathing techniques through his chair yoga practice. He experienced balance and harmony as he timed his breath with his heartbeat. He envisioned his heart reaching its natural rhythm, like a calming song, with each breath and expiration.

Robert's experience emphasizes the value of chair yoga's rhythmic breathing techniques. Focusing on your breath and slowly synchronizing it with your heart's beat will help you incorporate these exercises into your practice. Imagine the connection between your breath and heart, which will help you feel at ease and in good health. These exercises provide a space to connect with your body's natural rhythms in addition to supporting the health of your heart.

Mild Cardiovascular Exercises: Promoting Heart Health

Imagine your heart as a garden that benefits from gentle maintenance and needs care and attention to flourish. Chair yoga offers a road to heart-friendly movement with gentle cardiovascular movements that boost circulation without taxing your body.

Introduce yourself to Maria, a 70-year-old who thought cardiovascular activity was too taxing for her. She learned the transformational potential of gentle cardiovascular exercises through her chair yoga practice. She had a gradual awakening in her heart as a result of her seated marching, rhythmic foot tapping, and rhythmically raised arms. She pictured her heart being tended to and nurtured with each movement, just like a garden that had been soaked in sunlight.

Maria's experience highlights the value of low-impact cardiovascular exercises in chair yoga. Simple movements that encourage circulation can be incorporated into these exercises while you are seated. Think of your heart being fed with every action, promoting a feeling of vigor and wellbeing. These exercises provide a space to connect with your body's natural rhythms in addition to supporting heart health.

Flowing movement patterns: the heart's dance

Think of your body as a dancer, flowing gracefully through the waltz-like steps that respect the health of your heart. Chair yoga's flowing movement patterns offer a chance to embrace heart-friendly activity through a series of linked movements that encourage circulation without taxing your body.

Think about Grace, a 75-year-old who frequently thought that her heart needed to beat more quickly. She found the transformational power of flowing movement patterns through her chair yoga practice. She felt her heart responding with a sensation of awakening and vibrancy as she raised her arms high, gently stretched to the sides, and swayed. She visualized her heart dancing joyfully during each phase, like a lovely waltz.

Grace's experience highlights the value of chair yoga's fluid movement patterns. Connect these mild movements in a flowing way to create these sequences in your practice. Consider your heart as a dance that responds to each movement and improves circulation. These sequences provide a space to connect with your body's natural rhythms in addition to promoting heart health.

The Symphony of Well-Being: Mindful Cardio Awareness

Think of your consciousness as a conductor who coordinates the beat of your heart with the movements of your body. By creating a strong connection between your mind and heart, chair yoga offers a practice that encourages heart-friendly movement.

Take Samuel, a man of 72 who frequently experienced a sense of disconnection from his physical experiences. He became aware of the transforming potential of mindful cardiac awareness through his chair yoga practice. He envisioned his awareness guiding his motions in tune with his heartbeat as he concentrated on the beat of his own heart. He sensed his heart responding to his goal with each breath, like a symphony of contentment.

The transformational potential of attentive cardiac awareness in chair yoga is demonstrated by Samuel's experience. Practice each action while paying close attention to the rhythm of your heart. Imagine your awareness nourishing the health of your heart, allowing it to discover its own rhythm. This routine builds a strong bond between your mind and heart in addition to promoting heart health.

The Movement for Heart-Friendliness has a melody.

It is a celebration of life, connection, and wellbeing to embrace heart-friendly movement. The experiences of Grace, Robert, Maria, Grace, and Samuel highlight the positive effects of promoting heart health with low-impact cardio in chair yoga.

You are nourishing the health of your heart from the inside out as you practice rhythmic breathing exercises, accept light cardiovascular motions, flow through movement sequences, and create conscious cardiac awareness. Each practice becomes a way to a happier, more vibrant life, a stronger connection to your body, and a healthier heart.

In order to acknowledge your heart's beat, promote well-being, and encourage you to move through life with a sense of connection, energy, and joy, let's start a journey of heart-friendly movement through low-impact cardio for seniors in chair yoga.

Chapter 7

Relaxation and Stress Relief

Guided Relaxation Techniques

The ebb and flow of life's cycles that determine your well-being can be visualized as threads of tension and relaxation woven into a tapestry that is your body. With the help of guided relaxation techniques, chair yoga allows you to embrace the art of relaxing. This journey provides a break from the stresses of daily life and nurtures the renewal of your soul. Your body achieves equilibrium through the gradual practice of chair yoga, much as a tapestry finds its beauty in the interplay of colors.

Meet Susan, a 65-year-old who thought she couldn't afford to rest because of her hectic schedule. However, she discovered via her chair yoga practice that guided relaxation was more than just a break; it was a crucial component of self-care and wellbeing. She discovered that guided relaxation was a haven that refilled her spirit and added to her general vigor through calming words and deliberate breathing.

We'll examine the development of guided relaxation techniques in chair yoga in this chapter. We'll celebrate the power of relaxation that nourishes your spirit and inspires a sense of calm and regeneration via deep breathing techniques and mindfulness meditation.

Exercises for Deep Breathing: A Breath of Renewal

Think of your breath as a soothing river that welcomes calmness into your being while removing stress from it. Chair yoga's deep breathing techniques provide a way to intentionally breathe into relaxation, promoting calm and regeneration.

Take Emma, a 70-year-old who frequently experienced feelings of impending doom. She learned about the transforming power of deep breathing exercises through her chair yoga practice. She found that she could release tension by concentrating on her breath, taking deep breaths, and exhaling gently. She saw herself breathing out tension and allowing serenity to enter her body and mind with each breath.

Emma's experience highlights the value of chair yoga breathing techniques. Find a comfortable seat, pay attention to your breathing, and incorporate these exercises into your practice. Exhale slowly through your lips after taking a big breath through your nose and stretching your belly. Imagine the tension evaporating with each exhalation, making room for peace. These activities provide a peaceful inner haven in addition to relaxation.

A Journey Within: Mindfulness Meditation

Think of your mind as a huge, blank canvas where ideas drift in and out like passing clouds. Through the process of objectively examining your thoughts while doing chair yoga, you can find a technique to unwind that promotes present and tranquility.

Take David, a 72-year-old man whose worries frequently caused his mind to race. He learned the transformational power of mindfulness meditation through his chair yoga practice. He took a comfortable seat, closed his eyes, gently focused on his breath, and let his thoughts come and go without holding onto them. He visualized his thoughts as a calm lake that reflected the calmness within with each breath.

David's encounter highlights the value of attentive meditation in chair yoga. Find a calm area to sit comfortably and close your eyes so that you can incorporate this exercise into your daily routine. Keep your focus on your breathing while objectively observing your thoughts. Imagine that you are able to be present and at peace as your mind transforms into a calm zone.

Relaxing Muscles Progressively: Releasing Tension

Consider your body as a garden that occasionally needs sensitive care because to tension overgrowth. Through guided exercises that help you to tense and release various muscle groups, chair yoga provides a means to relax and promotes a feeling of physical and mental calm.

Meet James, a 68-year-old man who frequently held tension in his neck and shoulders. He learned about the transforming power of progressive muscular relaxation through his chair yoga practice. He felt a sensation of physical relief and mental calmness as he followed the guided instructions to tension and release his muscles. He visualized his body as a tranquil garden where stress dissolved away like falling leaves with each release.

The importance of progressive muscle relaxation in chair yoga is emphasized by James' experience. By locating a peaceful and cozy place to sit or lie down, include this practice into your daily routine. Follow the guided exercises to contract and release various muscle groups while visualizing the tension dissipating with each release. This exercise provides a place to let go of mental stress in addition to encouraging physical relaxation.

Guided visualization: A Renewal Journey

Imagine your mind as a blank canvas on which your imagination might create images of regeneration and peace. Through guided imaging exercises that take you to serene and revitalizing settings, guided visualization in chair yoga provides a means to relax and promotes a sense of peace and inner regeneration.

Take Sarah, a 75-year-old woman who frequently craved for little periods of freedom from life's obligations. She became aware of the transforming potential of guided imagery through her chair yoga practice. She let her mind transport her to a tranquil beach or a beautiful forest as she closed her eyes and followed the guided directions. She pictured herself immersing herself in the serenity of these settings with each vision, feeling a sense of calm and inner regeneration.

The relevance of guided visualization in chair yoga is demonstrated by Sarah's experience. By locating a peaceful and cozy place to sit or lie down, include this practice into your daily routine. As you listen to guided directions that take you through serene settings, close your eyes. Imagine your body and mind soaking up the peacefulness of these settings, giving you a sense of inner rebirth and peace.

The Relaxation Symphony

Techniques for guided relaxation are a celebration of calm, regeneration, and wellbeing. The experiences of Susan, Emma, David, James, and Sarah highlight the transforming impact of practicing chair yoga while relaxing.

You're entering a space of calm and regeneration that feeds your soul as you engage in deep breathing exercises, investigate mindfulness meditation, practice progressive muscle relaxation, and start guided visualizations. Every practice provides an opportunity to unwind, develop a closer relationship with your inner self, and experience calmness and peace.

So let's start our trip with guided relaxation methods in

Embraced by a soft hug of tranquility, chair yoga enables you to relax and revitalize while honoring your soul's need for rejuvenation.

Finding Inner Calm

Think of your mind as a wide desert, sometimes raging with ideas and in need of a tranquil oasis. Finding inner peace through chair yoga enables you to explore the oasis inside. This trip transcends the chaos of daily life and promotes the tranquility of your spirit. The mild chair yoga practice transforms your inner peace into a sanctuary, much like an oasis provides refuge in the desert.

Meet Lisa, a 60-year-old woman who thought inner peace was a pipe dream in the midst of her hectic schedule. Finding inner peace wasn't an escape, but a method to face problems in life with grace, as she discovered via her chair yoga practice. She discovered that inner peace was a path that contributed to her general well-being through mindfulness and intentional breathing.

We'll examine the process of obtaining inner peace through chair yoga in this chapter. We'll celebrate the power of presence that feeds your spirit and beckons a sense of calm and tranquility via mindfulness practices and breathing exercises.

Techniques for Mindfulness: Developing the Present Moment

Think of your awareness as a lantern, a light that illuminates the current moment and chases away distractions and worries. Chair yoga mindfulness practices provide a way to embrace the present moment with intention, building a sense of groundedness and tranquility, and helping one find inner quiet.

Take Emma, a 70-year-old who frequently found her thoughts straying to worries about the future. She learned about the transforming power of mindfulness through chair yoga. She experienced a sense of present and anchoring as she concentrated on the sensations of her breath, the sounds around her, or the sensation of her body in the chair. With each conscious breath, she visualized letting go of her worries and letting the present moment gently embrace her.

Emma's encounter highlights the value of mindfulness exercises in chair yoga. By settling into a comfortable seated position and focusing your mind on the present moment, you can include these strategies into your practice. Take note of your breath, your body's sensations, or the sounds in your environment. Think of your awareness as a light that leads you to a calm and present environment. These practices not only promote inner tranquility but also provide a haven of inner peace.

Exercises for Breathing: The Rhythm of Calm
Think of the rhythm of your breath as a calming song that nourishes your soul and calms your mind. By purposefully controlling your breath, breathing techniques in chair yoga provide a way to find inner serenity, encouraging a sensation of relaxation and tranquility.

Take David, a 72-year-old man who frequently felt trapped in a wave of ideas. He learned the transformational power of deliberate breathing through his chair yoga practice. He took a long breath in and let it out slowly, feeling the tension melt away. He visualized himself building a tranquil area within himself with each breath, like a peaceful oasis in the middle of the mental desert.

David's encounter highlights the value of breathing techniques in chair yoga. Find a comfortable seat, pay attention to your breathing, and incorporate these exercises into your practice. Take a big breath in with your nose and let it out gently through your mouth. Think of your breath as a song that calms your thoughts and gives you a feeling of peace and contentment. These activities not only promote inner peace but also provide a safe haven.

Connecting with Stability Through Grounding Visualization

Think of your body as a tree, firmly planted in the ground, strong, solid, and impervious to the raging winds. By visualizing yourself rooted in stability and connected to the Earth's energy, grounding imagery in chair yoga offers a route to discovering inner quiet, encouraging a sense of centeredness and tranquility.

Meet Michael, a 70-year-old who frequently felt paralyzed by the ambiguities of life. He learned about the transforming power of grounding imagery through his chair yoga practice. He closed his eyes and listened to the instructions, visualizing himself as a tree with deep, earth-bound roots. He experienced strength and solidity with each visualization, like a tree rooted to the ground.

Michael's experience highlights how crucial it is for chair yoga to ground visualization. By locating a peaceful and cozy place to sit or lie down, include this practice into your daily routine. Listen to the guided imagery as you close your eyes and visualize your body as a tree with roots reaching deep into the ground. Develop a sense of stability and inner peace by visualizing yourself as connected and rooted. This exercise not only promotes the health of your soul but also provides a place where you may feel safe inside.

Self-compassion and Affirmations: Growing Your Inner Garden

Think of your thoughts as seeds that can sprout into affirmations that promote your wellbeing and self-compassion. In chair yoga, affirmations and self-compassion create a route to inner peace by purposefully nurturing positive thoughts that promote peace and self-love.

Take Sarah, a 75-year-old who frequently battled self-criticism. She learned the transformational power of affirmations and self-compassion through her chair yoga practice.

She noticed a change in her inner dialogue when she recited peaceful affirmations like "I am calm," "I am at peace," or "I am worthy of love." Every time she said an affirmation, she visualized herself tending to her inner garden and cultivating kindness and self-love.

The importance of affirmations and self-compassion in chair yoga is demonstrated through Sarah's experience. By locating a peaceful and cozy place to sit or lie down, include this practice into your daily routine. Repeat encouraging statements to oneself, emphasizing kindness and self-love. Think of these affirmations as seeds that sprout inside a serene, rich landscape. This routine develops not only inner peace but also a place where your spirit may be cared for.

The Inner Calm Symphony
A celebration of presence, tranquility, and wellbeing is achieving inner peace. The

experiences of Lisa, Emma, David, Michael, and Sarah highlight the transforming impact of practicing chair yoga while experiencing inner stillness.

You're discovering a domain of calm that supports the health of your soul as you practice mindfulness techniques, breathing exercises, grounding visualization, and develop self-compassion through affirmations. Each practice develops into a path to inner peace, a closer relationship with your inner self, and a feeling of tranquility and harmony.

Let's therefore set off on a journey to discover inner peace through chair yoga—a trip that respects your soul's yearning for peace, promotes wellbeing, and encourages you to face

life's problems with a sense of grounded
presence and inner serenity.

Chapter 8

Tailoring Chair Yoga to Your Needs

Modifying Poses for Individual Comfort

Think of your practice as a blank canvas on which you can create your own unique work of movement and wellbeing. By adapting poses for personal comfort, chair yoga enables you to embrace your distinctive path—a journey that honors your body's requirements and supports your wellbeing in a way that is entirely your own. By making adjustments that respect your comfort and support your journey, you may personalize chair yoga in the same way that an artist adds their unique touch to a canvas.

Meet Alex, a 68-year-old who insisted on doing positions exactly as they were shown. However, he discovered a world where adjustments were welcomed and even encouraged through his chair yoga practice. He learned that altering poses allowed him to enjoy the advantages of each position in a way that felt cozy and supportive through attentive awareness and creative changes.

In this chapter, we'll examine the practice of chair yoga position modification for personal comfort. We'll celebrate the power of personalization that fosters your well-being and inspires a sense of empowerment and self-discovery, from paying attention to your body's signals to using props.

Knowing Your Body: Accessing the Wisdom
Within

Consider your body as a compass that directs
you in the direction of what feels good and
supportive. By paying attention to feelings,
discomfort, and signals that come during your
practice, chair yoga allows you to alter poses for
personal comfort.

Take Emma, a 70-year-old who frequently
experienced lower back stiffness while
performing specific poses. She learned the
transforming power of listening to her body
through her chair yoga practice. She was aware
of how her body was responding as she
performed various stances. She softly changed

her position or altered the movement to find a more comfortable alternative when a pose made her uncomfortable. She visualized her body's wisdom guiding her toward a practice that felt appropriate for her with each adjustment.

Emma's experience highlights how important it is to practice chair yoga while paying attention to your body. Pay close attention to any discomfort or sensations as you integrate this exercise into your daily routine. If a pose isn't comfortable, look into adjustments that fit your body's requirements. Consider the signals coming from your body as a compass that directs you to a practice that promotes your wellbeing.

Using Supporting Tools as Props

Consider your practice as a toolbox full of auxiliary items that can improve your experience and help you design a comfortable practice. By adding materials like blankets, pillows, or straps to the poses to provide support and stability, chair yoga poses can be altered for personal comfort.

Meet Sarah, a 75-year-old who frequently thought her flexibility was a limitation when stretching. She became aware of the transforming effect of employing props during her chair yoga practice. She discovered more comfort and stability in seated positions by placing a cushion beneath her hips. She slowly extended her reach with a strap whenever it became difficult to reach her feet. With each prop, she visualized adding greater levels of comfort and support to her practice.

Sarah's experience demonstrates the value of using props when doing chair yoga. Investigate the use of blankets, cushions, straps, and other comforting and supportive materials to incorporate this exercise into your daily routine. Think of these accessories as practice-enhancing tools that let you alter positions for improved comfort and stability. These tools not only improve your health but also provide you a sense of control over your practice.

Creative Modifications: Customizing Poses for You

Think of your practice as a piece of art that you can shape and modify to suit the requirements of your body. By experimenting with variations that feel right for you, creative adjustments in chair yoga offer a chance to change postures for individual comfort, encouraging a sense of self-discovery and ownership of your practice.

Take Michael, a 70-year-old whose range of motion frequently made it difficult for him to strike classic postures. He learned the transforming potential of creative modifications through his chair yoga practice. He came up with techniques to adapt movements that seemed approachable and pleasant rather than trying to replicate the precise stance. For example, when performing twists, he altered his arm positions, and when performing standing poses, he adopted a wider stance. He visualized himself creating a practice that embraced his individuality with each tweak.

Michael's experience highlights the value of inventive modifications in chair yoga. Investigate different variants of poses that feel good for your body as you include this practice into your daily routine. Consider your practice as a blank canvas that you may customize to your preferences in order to encourage self-discovery and creativity. These changes not only improve your health but also provide you the chance to create a practice that is uniquely yours.

The Crowning Glory of Your Practice
Pose adjustments are a celebration of one's own self-awareness, community, and empowerment. The experiences of Alex, Emma, Sarah, and

Michael show the transformational impact of accepting modifications in chair yoga.

You are producing an original work of movement and wellbeing as you pay attention to your body's signals, use props for support, experiment with creative changes, and adjust postures to your comfort. Each adjustment opens the door to a practice that is more comfortable, a closer relationship with your body, and a sense of empowerment and self-discovery.

Therefore, let's begin the path of adapting chair yoga postures for personal comfort—a journey that respects your body's knowledge, promotes wellbeing, and invites you to create your own unique movement and self-expression.

Addressing Specific Health Concerns

Think of your practice as a garden, a place where you may nurture wellbeing and tenderly attend to individual needs. A journey that customizes your practice to meet your body's specific needs, chair yoga enables you to nurture your wellbeing by addressing specific health conditions. Through chair yoga, you may tend to your body in the same way as a gardener would to various plants with specific care, promoting balance and energy.

Introducing Emily, a 72-year-old who felt her health issues prevented her from practicing yoga. However, she discovered a world where she could modify her practice to suit her needs through her chair yoga adventure. She found that chair yoga was a method to enhance her well-being and add to her general vigor through targeted motions and gentle exercises.

We'll look at how to use chair yoga to specifically address various health issues in this chapter. We'll celebrate the power of adjusting your practice to suit your body's requirements, from treating arthritis to easing back pain, and we'll encourage a sense of empowerment and healing.

Managing Arthritis: Adopting Gentle Movement

Think of your joints as hinges that benefit from gentle movements that offer support and pain alleviation. By adding mild exercises that encourage joint mobility and reduce pain, chair yoga offers a means to address arthritis.

Consider David, a 70-year-old with arthritis whose knees were frequently stiff. He discovered the transformational power of soft movements through his chair yoga practice. He discovered that he could gently move his joints without increasing pain by doing exercises like ankle circles, wrist rotations, and sitting twists. He pictured his joints getting the attention they required with each movement, like an efficient machine.

David's experience highlights the importance of managing arthritis in chair yoga. Include light exercises that focus on the troubled joints in your routine. Consider these motions as supportive and caring gestures that promote joint mobility and reduce pain. In addition to nourishing your joints, these exercises also provide you a feeling of relief and authority over your practice.

Relieving Back Pain While Promoting Spinal Health

Think of your spine as a pillar of strength that requires stability and support to remain healthy. By incorporating poses and motions that promote spinal health and ease discomfort, chair yoga offers a technique to address back pain.

Introducing Sarah, a 65-year-old with chronic lower back discomfort. She learned the transformational effect of poses that focused on her spine through her chair yoga practice. She discovered that she could foster the health of her back while avoiding tension by doing mild twists, forward folds, and seated stretches. She visualized her spine gaining strength and flexibility with each motion, like a strong pillar of support.

Sarah's experience demonstrates the value of chair yoga for treating back pain. Include postures and exercises that focus on your spine and ease pain throughout your practice. Think of these motions as supportive and restorative actions that promote spinal health and wellbeing. In addition to strengthening your back, these exercises give you a feeling of relief and authority over your practice.

Reducing Stress: Promoting Calm and Relaxation

Consider your mind as a tranquil body of water that occasionally becomes agitated by stress and requires a calming breeze. By mixing mindfulness practices and relaxation exercises that promote calmness and peace, chair yoga provides a method for dealing with stress.

Take Emma, a 68-year-old who frequently felt overburdened by the demands of daily life. She learned the transformational power of mindfulness and relaxation through her chair yoga practice. She discovered that she could incorporate peaceful moments into her work by using deep breathing techniques, guided meditations, and progressive muscular relaxation. She visualized her stress evaporating with each breath, like waves on a pond.

Emma's experience highlights how important stress management is in chair yoga. Include mindfulness practices and calming exercises in your routine to promote peace and tranquility. Think of these routines as little periods of relaxation that nurture your wellbeing and provide you a place to let stress go. In addition to nourishing your mind, these practices also give you a calm sense of empowerment.

Balance Improvement: Promoting Stability

Think of your body like a gracefully swaying tree that occasionally needs help to stand tall and powerful. By incorporating postures and motions that promote stability and enhance equilibrium, chair yoga offers a way to address balance concerns.

Meet Michael, a 75-year-old who frequently experienced balance issues as a result of aging. He learned the transforming potential of balance-enhancing moves through his chair yoga practice. He discovered that he could gently test his stability while seated by performing exercises like leg lifts, ankle circles, and sat balances. He visualized his body finding a rooted sense of solidity with each movement, like a tree securely planted in the ground.

Michael's experience serves as a demonstration of the value of balance improvement in chair yoga. Include exercises that will make it difficult for you to maintain your balance while seated.

Consider these motions as displays of strength and support that promote equilibrium and stability. These movements not only improve your balance but also give you a sense of control and assurance in your abilities.

Your Individual Wellness Garden

Taking care of certain health issues is a celebration of self-care, assistance, and empowerment. The experiences of Emily, David, Sarah, Emma, and Michael demonstrate the transforming potential of customizing your chair yoga practice.

You are attending to your body's particular demands and creating a sense of balance and energy as you manage arthritis, alleviate back pain, reduce stress, improve balance, and deal with other health issues. Each adjustment opens the door to a practice that is more personalized to your needs, a closer relationship with your body's wisdom, and a feeling of empowerment and healing.

So let's begin the adventure of using chair yoga to treat certain health issues; a path that respects the individuality of your body, promotes wellbeing, and invites you to grow your own personal garden of support and wellness.

Chapter 9

Creating a Consistent Practice

Establishing a 10-Minute Daily Routine

Imagine your day as a blank canvas on which you can paint vibrant, happy strokes in just ten minutes. By creating a 10-minute routine, chair yoga welcomes you to infuse your daily life with brightness. This path respects your time, cares for your body, and invites a daily practice that fits easily into your schedule. Your 10-minute chair yoga session can infuse your day with energy, much as a dawn offers a burst of light to the globe.

Meet Ava, a 65-year-old woman who felt she didn't have time to practice yoga. However, she discovered via her chair yoga adventure that all it took was 10 minutes to reap the rewards of a regular regimen. She learned that a quick practice could produce a ripple of well-being that lasted throughout her day through certain positions and deliberate breathing.

We'll look at how to create a 10-minute chair yoga routine in this chapter. We'll celebrate the power of a regular practice that adds brightness to your life, from developing a routine that works with your schedule to choosing postures that energize your body.

Creating Your Space: A Haven of Calm

Think of your practice area as a sacred haven where you can retreat to achieve peace and concentration. By making sure you have a cozy and welcoming location to practice in, creating your space for chair yoga lays the groundwork for your 10-minute routine.

A 70-year-old man named James set aside a spot in his living room for his daily chair yoga practice. He made a tranquil haven out of the area by adding a cozy chair, a mat, and a plush cushion. Every day as he reached this area, he visualized entering a realm of relaxation and renewal.

James's experience emphasizes how important it is to make your own space when practicing chair yoga. Locate a spot in your house where you can comfortably practice. Set up a chair, a mat, and any other props you might require in the area. Think of this area as a tranquil retreat where you are encouraged to fully devote yourself to your practice.

Choosing Poses: A Symphony of Motion

Think of your practice as a symphony, a flowing progression of postures that enlivens your body and spirit. By choosing moves that target particular parts of your body and stimulate your vigor, chair yoga poses help to structure your 10-minute program.

Emma, a 68-year-old woman, started her 10-minute workout with some gentle stretching and deep breathing techniques. She then performed balance-improving positions and a quick relaxing exercise. She pictured her body waking up and becoming a symphony of movement with each stance.

Emma's experience demonstrates the value of choosing positions when practicing chair yoga. Pick poses that fit the demands and objectives of your body. Warm up with moderate stretches in the beginning, including poses that target certain issues, and finish with a relaxing method. Imagine your daily routine as a symphony that nourishes and energizes your body.

The Setting Intention: A Guideline

Think of your practice as a trip that you set out on with purpose and intention. By focusing your attention and giving your practice purpose, setting intention during chair yoga gives your 10-minute routine direction.

Take David, a 72-year-old who started each practice with the straightforward goal of cultivating calm and wellbeing. He closed his eyes and said aloud his purpose as he sat in his chair. He visualized his aim as a light that guided him through his practice with each breath.

David's experience highlights the value of intention-setting in chair yoga. Consider taking a moment to create an intention before starting your routine. It could be to promote calmness, take care of your body, or just to savor the present. Think of this objective as a beacon that gives your practice direction and significance.

10-Minute Routine: A Radiance Blast

Think of your practice as a momentary, yet potent, burst of well-being that brightens your day. Your daily focus shifts to your 10-minute chair yoga session, where you can lose yourself in movement, breathing, and self-care.

Meet Michael, a 75-year-old who developed a morning ritual that lasted 10 minutes. He started by taking a few slow, deep breaths to ground himself and then gently stretching to awaken his body. He included balance-enhancing poses and finished with a quick relaxation practice. He saw injecting his day with a boost of energy and well-being with each workout.

Michael's experience demonstrates the value of a 10-minute chair yoga program. Set out a certain period each day that works with your schedule for practice. Start with a few slow, deep breaths to ground yourself, then move through a series of positions that correspond to the demands of your body, and finish with a relaxation method. Think of your daily ritual as a flash of radiance that gives your day life and self-care.

Throughout Your Day, Radiance

Setting up a chair yoga routine for 10 minutes is a celebration of time, energy, and self-care. The experiences of Ava, James, Emma, David, and Michael show the transforming effect of incorporating a brief practice into daily life.

You're producing a flash of radiance that improves your wellbeing and sets the tone for your day as you prepare your space, choose positions, set purpose, and immerse yourself in your 10-minute ritual. Each practice turns into a means of sustaining life, a time for self-care, and a place to care for your body and spirit.

So let's start a 10-minute chair yoga routine that respects your time, promotes wellbeing, and asks you to add a dose of radiance and self-care to your day.

Staying Motivated and Inspired

Imagine your drive as a flame, a burst of inspiration that fuels your resolve and keeps you going. A path that honors your commitment, feeds your passion, and invites a consistent practice that changes with you, chair yoga urges you to feed your inner fire by remaining inspired and motivated. Your inner fire can enlighten your chair yoga journey with zeal and dedication, just as a flame illuminates the darkness.

Meet Olivia, a 70-year-old who thought it was difficult to stay motivated. However, she discovered a world where remaining motivated was possible through her chair yoga adventure. She learned that her inner fire could burn brightly through thoughtful techniques and original thinking, giving her practice fresh life.

We'll look at how to stay inspired and motivated throughout your chair yoga experience in this chapter. We'll celebrate the importance of creating an inner fire that moves your practice ahead with enthusiasm and devotion, from setting goals to investigating new variants.

Setting Objectives: A North Star

Think of your practice as a journey—a road you travel while maintaining a firm sense of direction. By outlining your objectives and aiming towards significant benchmarks, setting goals for chair yoga gives your trip a North Star.

Consider Alex, a 68-year-old man who wanted to become more flexible. He added particular poses and stretches that were targeted at his tight regions into his practice. He experienced a sense of advancement and accomplishment after every drill, as if he were getting closer to his North Star.

The importance of having goals when practicing chair yoga is highlighted by Alex's experience. Decide what it is that you hope to accomplish via your practice, whether it is more flexibility, less stress, or better balance. Your program should include focused poses and your aim should be broken down into doable increments. Think of your objective as a North Star that will help you go with direction and vigor.

An Artistic Tapestry: Exploring Variations

Think of your practice as a tapestry—a blank canvas on which you can weave your distinct creativity and discover new possibilities. By incorporating unique ideas into your routine and stimulating a sense of novelty and curiosity, experimenting with different chair yoga variations offers a method to stay inspired and motivated.

Meet Sarah, a 65-year-old who enjoyed modifying and attempting new stances. She frequently experimented with fresh versions rather than adhering to the same pattern. She experimented with various breathing exercises, made imaginative changes, and even inserted soft music into her routine. She experienced a rush of exhilaration and a fresh feeling of inspiration with each investigation.

Sarah's experience demonstrates the value of researching different chair yoga modifications. Give yourself permission to experiment with new poses, alter your routine's motions, and add new components. Think of your practice as a blank canvas on which you can paint your imagination and curiosity. These changes encourage inspiration and motivation while also keeping your practice novel.

The Gift of Presence: Mindful Practice

Think of your practice as a present that you carefully open with mindfulness and intention.

By encouraging you to completely engage with each movement, breath, and sensation, mindful chair yoga offers a means to maintain motivation and inspiration while building a sense of present and connection.

Take 75-year-old Michael, who adopted mindfulness in his practice. Instead of hurrying through his routine, he focused entirely on each moment. He focused on his breathing, enjoyed the feelings in his body, and stayed in the present. He experienced a strong sense of connection and rekindled enthusiasm for his practice with each breath.

Michael's experience highlights the value of mindful chair yoga practice. With intention and mindfulness, approach each practice. Immerse yourself in the present moment, pay attention to your breathing, and concentrate on your body's sensations. Think of your practice as a present that you open with mindfulness and appreciation. This thoughtful method keeps you interested while also inspiring creativity and motivation.

Journaling and Introspection: A Source of Wisdom

Think of your practice as a route where you can discover new perspectives and reflections as you go. With the ability to record your accomplishments, experiences, and thoughts, journaling and reflection in chair yoga give you a means to stay motivated and inspired while building a sense of self-awareness and growth.

Meet Emma, a 68-year-old who chronicled her chair yoga adventure in a journal. She kept a journal after every practice, writing about how she felt, the difficulties she faced, and any new insights she had gained. She marveled at her development and tenacity as she read back over her notebook throughout time. She experienced a burst of inspiration to keep up her practice with each reflection.

Emma's story demonstrates the value of journaling and introspection in chair yoga. Keep a journal where you can record your ideas, encounters, and development. Write about your experience doing chair yoga, any new insights you had, and how you feel about it now. Think of your notebook as a source of wisdom that you may tap into for inspiration and motivation.

Fire Up Your Inner Flame

Maintaining inspiration and motivation is a celebration of commitment, imagination, and attentiveness. The stories of Olivia, Alex, Sarah, Michael, and Emma show the transforming potential of developing an inner fire that motivates your chair yoga journey.

You're kindling your inner fire and bringing enthusiasm and commitment to your practice as you create goals, investigate variants, practice mindfully, journal, and reflect. Every exercise becomes a source of inspiration, an area for creativity, and a journey toward self-awareness.

Let's set out on a journey to maintain inspiration and motivation in your chair yoga practice—a journey that respects your dedication, promotes wellness, and asks you to develop an inner fire that lights your way with passion and vitality.

Chapter 10

Chair Yoga Beyond the Mat

Integrating Mindfulness into Daily Life

Think of your life as a tapestry made up of moments, with each thread standing for a chance to bring mindfulness into your everyday activities. The practice of chair yoga encourages you to embrace mindful living, a path that celebrates the importance of being present, strengthens your relationship with others, and encourages you to appreciate each moment as it comes. By incorporating mindfulness into your daily activities, you may create a masterpiece of mindful living, just like an artist does with each brushstroke.

Introducing Sophia, a 72-year-old who thought mindfulness only applied to her own practice. However, she discovered a world where practicing mindfulness was a way of life that permeated every area of her day through her chair yoga adventure. She found that every moment had the potential for presence and connection through mindful eating, walking, and even conversation.

We'll talk about how to incorporate mindfulness into your daily life in this chapter. We'll celebrate the power of developing awareness that enhances experiences and encourages a closer connection with the environment around you, from mindful dining to mindful exercise.

Savoring each bite while eating mindfully

Consider your meal to be an orchestra of flavors—a feast for the senses that demands your undivided attention. Savoring each bite while eating mindfully allows you to incorporate mindfulness into your daily life and develop a greater appreciation for the food you are given.

Consider James, a 65-year-old who frequently ate quickly without fully appreciating his meals. He learned that mindful eating has the power to transform through his chair yoga practice. He started by pausing to consider the flavors, textures, and scents of his cuisine. He chewed deliberately with each bite, savoring the flavors and engrossing himself in the moment. He visualized his body receiving not only nourishment but also a sense of gratitude with each thoughtful meal.

James' experience highlights how important mindful eating is in chair yoga. Take a time to curiously inspect your food as you are eating. Chew gently and enjoy every bite, savoring the flavors and textures as you go. Think of your meal as a harmonious performance of nourishment that you enjoy mindfully and with gratitude.

Moving mindfully: Being Present in Motion

Think of your body as an instrument of awareness—a graceful, purposeful vehicle that propels you through life. By incorporating awareness into your movements, mindful movement offers a means to incorporate mindfulness into your daily life and promote a stronger bond between your body and mind.

A 68-year-old woman named Emma practices mindful movement throughout her day. She handled every task with presence and intention, whether she was walking, cleaning, or gardening. She concentrated on her bodily feelings, her breathing pattern, and the precision of her motions. She visualized herself walking through life with ease and awareness with each step.

The relevance of focused movement in chair yoga is demonstrated by Emma's experience. Approaching your everyday activities with presence and attention will help. Pay attention to the way your body feels, how you breathe, and how well you move. Consider every move as a chance to navigate life with purpose and elegance.

Breathing mindfully: The Foundation of Presence

Think of your breath as an anchor, a constant source of concentration that maintains you in the here and now. Using your breath as a tool to create present and serenity, mindful breathing offers a means to incorporate mindfulness into your daily life.

Think of David, a 70-year-old who made mindful breathing a part of his daily routine. He stopped periodically throughout the day to pay attention to his breath. He allowed his breath to lead him to the present moment as he paid attention to the sensation of each inhalation and exhalation. He visualized himself focusing on the present moment with each focused breath.

David's experience highlights how important conscious breathing is in chair yoga. Take breaks during the day to reflect on your breath. Allow your breath to center you in the here and now as you pay attention to how you feel as you inhale and exhale. Consider your breath as an anchor that helps you stay centered and relaxed.

Mindful Conversations: Present-Day Listening

Consider your interactions as dances of connection where you may both hear and be heard completely. By actively listening and speaking during a discussion, you may incorporate mindfulness into your daily life and strengthen your relationships with others.

Meet Sophia, a woman of 72 who brought mindfulness to her interactions. She worked on her active listening skills when conversing with people, paying close attention to their words, tones, and body language. She also used deliberate speech, carefully selecting her words, and gave herself time to think before responding. She visualized herself creating connections and understanding through each thoughtful interaction.

The relevance of focused discourse in chair yoga is demonstrated by Sophia's experience. Engage in active listening during conversations by concentrating entirely on the speaker. Be careful while choosing your words, speak with intention, and give yourself permission to reply in the same manner. Consider your interactions with others as conscious, present dances of connection.

A Life Illuminated by Presence: Mindful Moments By incorporating mindfulness
Your everyday activities are a celebration of awareness, connection, and presence. The stories of Sophia, James, Emma, David, and countless others show the transformative power of living mindfully.

You are weaving awareness into the fabric of your daily experiences as you practice mindful eating, embrace mindful activity, nurture mindful breathing, partake in mindful discussions, and appreciate mindful moments. Every moment becomes a chance for the present, a chance to strengthen your ties to the people and things around you, and an invitation to lead a life that is enlightened by mindfulness.

Let's therefore start the journey of incorporating mindfulness into daily life—a trip that values each moment, cultivates your relationship with the outside world, and asks you to enrich your experiences with the richness of presence and awareness.

Sharing the Benefits with Others

Think of your practice as a gift you may give to others as you share the joy of chair yoga with the world. Chair yoga enables you to adopt the position of a beacon—a leader who shows people around you the way to wellbeing. Sharing the advantages of chair yoga with others makes you an inspiration, improving not only your own well-being but also the lives of people you come in contact with.

Meet Ethan, a 68-year-old who found delight in teaching chair yoga to his neighborhood. He thought the advantages of chair yoga were too valuable to keep to himself. He taught others about the practice's transforming impact through gentle classes at community events and senior centers in the area. His sharing journey turned into a lighthouse of happiness, illuminating the lives of everyone he touched.

This chapter will examine the technique of educating people about the advantages of chair yoga. We'll celebrate the power of becoming a source of well-being and a mentor for a healthier, more fulfilling life, whether it be teaching others or motivating loved ones.

Leading Classes: An Inspirational Source

Think of your practice as a spark that you can spread to inspire others to go on their own path to wellbeing. By guiding participants through the practice, developing a sense of community, and allowing them to set out on their own road of transformation, instructors of chair yoga sessions can spread the benefits of the practice to others.

Take Olivia, a 70-year-old who earned her chair yoga certification. She started teaching chair yoga courses at her neighborhood community center and encouraging people to join her. She saw her pupils achieve new levels of strength and flexibility via gentle direction and considerate adjustments. She visualized herself igniting a flame of happiness in the hearts of her students with each lesson.

Olivia's experience highlights the value of instructing chair yoga lessons. If you feel inspired, think about teaching chair yoga or teaching it to others in your neighborhood. Help them through the exercise, provide adjustments, and promote a sense of camaraderie. Consider each lesson as a spark that ignites happiness in the lives of your students.

Motivating Family and Friends: A Ripple of Well-Being

Think of your practice as a ripple: a little deed that sends ripples of good throughout the world. By introducing them to the practice, fostering their well-being, and enticing them to embrace self-care, encouraging loved ones to try chair yoga is a method to spread awareness of its advantages.

Meet Ava, a 65-year-old who taught chair yoga to her family. She started by teaching her grandchildren some basic stretches and breathing techniques. Chair yoga eventually became a family tradition as her children and grandkids joined her in her daily ritual. Ava thought of herself as creating a positive ripple in the lives of her loved ones with each shared moment.

The lesson learned from Ava's experience is the importance of encouraging loved ones to try chair yoga. Talk about easy stretches and exercises with your family and friends. Encourage them to take up chair yoga and join you in your practice. Think of each shared moment as a ripple of happiness that improves the lives of the people you care about.

Supporting Community Wellness: A Shared Vision

Think of your practice as a bridge, connecting others who might not have otherwise heard of chair yoga to its advantages. By working with neighborhood organizations, senior centers, or health fairs to bring chair yoga to various groups, supporting wellness in your community offers a chance to spread the advantages to a wider audience.

Meet Ethan, a 68-year-old who created chair yoga sessions with the help of his community center. By reaching those who might not have access to such techniques, he saw the opportunity to have a bigger influence. He taught chair yoga to elders, caregivers, and others with restricted mobility with the help of neighborhood organizations. He pictured himself as a bridge linking people to the delight of well-being with each lesson.

Ethan's story highlights how important it is to promote wellbeing in your community. Offer chair yoga classes in conjunction with community organizations, senior centers, or health fairs. Reach out to various groups and explain the advantages of the practice to them. Consider yourself a conduit for introducing people to the transforming potential of chair yoga.

Making a Ripple Effect of Well-Being

Giving others access to chair yoga's advantages is a celebration of kindness, empathy, and inspiration. The stories of Ethan, Olivia, Ava, and numerous others show the transformative potential of shining as a light of happiness for people around you.

You are spreading happiness, nourishing lives, and expanding the joy of chair yoga when you teach classes, encourage loved ones, promote wellness in your neighborhood, and share the practice with others.

So let's set off on a journey to spread the joy of chair yoga, illuminating lives with inspiration and optimism as we do so. This journey respects the gift of wellbeing, encourages connection, and invites you to share the joy of chair yoga with others.

Conclusion

Celebrating Your Journey to Senior Wellness

Think of your trip as a constellation, a group of stars that show you the way to radiant health. The practice of chair yoga encourages you to accept your path with appreciation, paying tribute to the actions you've taken, the learnings you've made, and the changes you've gone through. As you come to the end of this manual, keep in mind that your journey is a continuing experience that is intertwined with opportunities for development, self-discovery, and happiness.

Meet Grace, a 75-year-old chair yoga enthusiast who set out on her adventure with curiosity and tenacity. She started out skeptical but soon became enthralled by the soothing stretches, deliberate breathing, and empowering poses. She experienced a fresh sense of connection with her body, peace, and vigor with each practice. Grace's experience served as a testament to the chair yoga's transformational potential and encouraged her to joyfully celebrate her recovery.

You've now had a chance to delve into the many facets of chair yoga, a kind of exercise that goes beyond simple physical poses and incorporates mindfulness, balance, community, and self-care. Your journey has been one of exploration, progress, and celebration—from comprehending the advantages to developing mindful moments.

Think about the moments that stand out as you reflect on your journey: the times you discovered a new stretch that made you smile, the times your breath synchronized with your movements, and the times you felt a profound connection to both yourself and the world around you.

Consider these experiences as stars in your constellation—a group of brilliant recollections that point you in the direction of ongoing wellbeing. Every minute of your journey adds to the fabric of your life, just as every star adds to the beauty of the night sky.

Taking Radiant Wellness to Heart

Your experience with chair yoga is a celebration of empowerment, self-care, and change. The experiences of Grace, you, and countless others highlight the transforming potential of chair yoga—a routine that promotes health in body, mind, and spirit.

Keep practicing self-compassion as you proceed on your journey. You might alternate between days of quiet, meditative practice and days when you push yourself to try new poses. Each movement, breath, and stride you take is a gift to yourself on your journey to radiant wellbeing and a life full of energy.

Continue to embrace your adventure with an open heart as you go forward. Each exercise should serve as a reminder of your inner strength, devotion to self-care, and dedication to wellbeing. Celebrate the accomplishments, calming, and joyful moments that chair yoga has brought into your life.

You too have the chance to design a path brimming with self-discovery, growth, and radiant wellness, just as Grace was enthralled by the transforming power of chair yoga. Your path is like a constellation, a road map to your own happiness that is only waiting to be discovered and honored.

As you proceed with the transformative adventure of chair yoga, may your journey be radiant, your well-being be bountiful, and your spirit be lifted.